Shy No More!

MASTERING THE ART OF SEDUCTION AND SOCIAL SKILLS

Giovanni Amato

This book is dedicated to all the women in my life,
both those from the past and those in the present. I
want to thank each and every one of you, for thanks
to you, I have learned so much about life and you have
made me who I am. Without you, I wouldn't be here
now writing this book, nor would I have known cities,
countries, and many other facets of life. You have
also made me knowledgeable about the principles of
seduction that I am now trying to convey in this book.
Each of you is unique and wonderful. Thank you very
much for making me a better person. You know I am a
free spirit, but I always remember you.

CONTENTS

INTRODUCTION

This is not just any book about seduction and personal development. It is a book born from over ten years of experience and knowledge in the field of seduction, personal development, and social skills. It emerges after having helped many men who, like you, were also shy and insecure, but thanks to the principles of seduction outlined here, they managed to achieve their goals and put an end to their suffering and discomfort, becoming true seducers.

This is a book in which I will guide you through the challenging path of overcoming shyness to become a seducer, a new alpha male, a confident, decisive man, and the best version of yourself.

The goal of this book is to bring out your full potential, focusing on naturalness, reflection, self-inspection, and self-discovery. By the end of the reading, you will be aware of your weaknesses to improve them and your strengths to apply them and enhance all aspects of your personal, emotional, and seductive life, aiming to bring out your best version, leaving behind shyness, mental baggage, and fears that hinder your progress in your social and emotional life.

I warn you, this is not a magical book or a step-by-step guide with invented techniques for picking up women. Instead, it is a book where I will invite you to discover your own essence, to discover yourself, to trust yourself, to bring out your best version, and to succeed in your future relationships.

This is not a book to read in one afternoon, as it contains very important principles of seduction, narrated through real stories, which you must internalize and chew thoroughly to digest them correctly. Otherwise, they may get stuck and cause indigestion.

So I recommend that you take the reading seriously, read it slowly, go back and read it again, do the exercises I propose in each chapter with the utmost sincerity, but don't forget the most important thing: take action. Don't just limit yourself to reading it, because reading without taking action will get you nowhere, so you'll waste your time and your money.

So if you're eager to make a radical change in your life, if you want to start having casual encounters, or if you want to start having a successful relationship with the girl you like, or if you want to go from being shy to becoming the seducer you've always wanted to be... without a doubt, this book is for you.

But listen up! Before you start reading it, I warn you that... if you don't first commit to making a change in your life, I won't be able to do anything for you, because in this beautiful life we live, nothing is achieved without commitment, effort, and suffering.

Therefore, I'm not going to promise you an easy path of unicorns, fairies, and fantasies, or immediate success. On the contrary, after putting the principles written here into practice, you're going to fail a lot, and then even more, but after getting up and learning from your mistakes, I promise you that you'll become the seducer you desire. As long as you're willing to pay the price of commitment, responsibility, effort, and change.

Are you ready to start this journey, make a change in your life, bring out your best version, and become that confident, successful, and seductive person you've always wanted to be? Let's get started!

BEFORE STARTING

5 keys to reading this book

I would like to give you some guidelines on how to read this book properly. You can follow them or not, it's up to you, but I think they are very important guidelines not only for reading this book, but for any self-help book you may want to read in the future.

1. Approach with an open mind. Be receptive to change, let yourself be advised, and always draw your own conclusions from what is written here. Don't take everything I say as gospel. Embrace uncertainty, accept your weaknesses and flaws. Work on improving them, focus on being your best self, and internalize the keys to seduction.

2. Do a quick read. Capture the key points and assimilate the content. Then, do a second, deeper reading, extracting the principles found here, underlining the phrases

or words that are key to you, and making notes on the pages about the reflections, ideas, or solutions that come to mind.

3. This is more of a suggestion, in which I invite you to share this book with a friend who is in the same situation as you, so that you can motivate each other and help each other with the learning process. Perhaps someone interprets something differently and you can discuss it together and reflect on it. Two minds are better than one, that's a fact.

4. Keep a notebook, either on your phone or on paper, whichever you prefer. The important thing is that when you are putting into action what you've learned in this book, you jot down your thoughts, successful or failed interactions, and try to draw your own conclusions, based on what you've learned from your own experience and from this book. This way, you'll reinforce what you've learned in a deeper way, which will make it easier for you to become a new seducer.

5. Return to this book and reread it whenever you need to. It's no secret that humans tend to forget what we learned if we let it slip for a while. As the author of my previous book, "Seductive Mindset," I still

reread it from time to time to remind myself of what I wrote back then, especially when I need motivation or inspiration. When you feel uncertain, pick up the book again and get motivated once more.

If you decide to follow the five pieces of advice I give you, you will be able to make the most of the content found here. Only in this way, in my personal opinion, will you be able to get the most out of this manuscript and achieve the greatest benefit from it. Remember never to forget to put everything you have learned into practice, to take the reading very seriously, and to do all the exercises proposed.

Having said all this, I believe you are now ready to begin reading, so your path to change is about to begin. Start believing in yourself; change is possible. Happy reading!

*"As a key opens many doors, so does
a seducer." - Giovanni Amato*

PART I:

The Mindset Shift,
From Shy to Seducer

DECODING THE ORIGINS OF YOUR SHYNESS

CHAPTER I

Everyone knows that there are people who are naturally extroverted, it's obvious, but if you've decided to get this book, then it's probably not your case. Therefore, you'll need to put in effort and work to change your condition.

I imagine you're more of a shy and insecure person who wants to stop being so, and we'll take advantage of that drive and motivation you have for change to make a difference in your shy condition. Because as you already know, everything in life can be changed if you take action and have the courage to do so.

So, can shyness be overcome? Absolutely, it may be easier or harder depending on the type of person you are, but it can definitely be changed, and you can go from being shy to becoming a seducer.

To understand shyness in its nature, let's see what types of shyness exist, their reasons, and later we'll see how to resolve them. But first, let's understand and comprehend what your problem is. Let's look at the cases of shyness:

1. **Chronic Shyness**: This type of shyness is characterized by total lack of self-confidence, and lacking confidence, we transmit this to every aspect of life, so everything generates fear and distrust. We could say it's the worst form of shyness, the most complicated, and the one that will require the most effort to overcome.

2. **Situational Shyness**: In this case, we would talk more about social anxiety, which could be initiating a first conversation with a stranger, attending an event, etc. Ultimately, it's the most common of all and therefore the easiest to overcome.

3. **Affective Shyness**: This type of shyness arises in the romantic or sexual realm. It could be the fear of expressing your feelings, showing affection, or touching the other person. In short, it's the fear of engaging in any kind of contact with the gender you're attracted to.

4. **Cognitive Shyness**: Cognitive shyness refers to social anxiety that arises in situ-

ations requiring cognitive skills, such as teamwork, problem-solving, or decision-making.

Now that you're clear about the types of shyness that exist, I hope you've realized which one is yours. It could be one, two, or even all of them. The important thing here is that you're honest with yourself, understand what your problem is, and be open to changing it.

Let's get to the important part because I'm sure you're wondering, "This is all well and good, but what's the solution?" Perfect, let's get to it, my friend. But first, let me tell you my personal story to motivate you and help you understand the principles for overcoming shyness.

From as far back as I can remember until my twenties, I had always been a very shy person. I was afraid of everything—expressing my opinion, talking to strangers, and the idea of starting a conversation with a woman or anyone unknown terrified me. When the occasion arose, I stuttered and usually turned as red as a tomato. And since I'm naturally red-haired to begin with, you can imagine the scene... It was quite a spectacle, as you can imagine.

Clearly, all of this frustrated me and occupied my mind a lot. You could say I wasn't happy because I felt that shyness was a burden in my life from which I couldn't break free, hindering my full development in any aspect of my life. Fortunately, I was aware of all this, and whenever I could, I reflected on the problem. However, I couldn't find a feasible solution. I lied to myself (out of cowardice) that maybe that's just how I was, that my natural condition was to be fearful, shy, and unable to talk to a woman. Of course, all of this was unfounded self-deception I imposed on myself, out of fear of facing reality and fear of stepping out of my "comfort zone." Which was nothing more than a cold and uncomfortable cave in the middle of Antarctica. Unfortunately, I still didn't know any other reality, so I clung to it as if there were no other alternative.

Fortunately, this changed one day. It wasn't overnight by any means; it was a slow journey and process, but I changed. The reason was that I realized the problem stemmed from how I was talking to myself and how I was viewing the world. I didn't accept myself as I was. My internal dialogues were all negative—I didn't like myself, saw myself as unattractive, believed I was insecure. Ultimately, I wasn't saying anything positive to myself, so I had fears and limiting beliefs that I had imposed on myself. Moreover, my worldview was entirely negative, so I thought everything was against me and that I was living in a hostile world where I would be judged for anything that went wrong. Again, it was a childish schoolboy thought that was difficult to overcome, but as you can see, it was a completely irrational thought, and fortunately, I was starting to become aware of it.

I realized all this simply by observing. I saw friends who were able to talk, flirt with women, go on dates, while I couldn't. I always asked myself, "What was wrong with me that made me different from them? Am I less? Do I lack courage? Is it all mental? How can I overcome it? Why am I shy, and they're not?"

The conclusion was that I was the problem. I was my own worst enemy at that moment, and it was solely up to me to turn things around, so I did. I decided to grab hold of the reins of my life and make a change until I became what I am now —a writer, a traveler, a partygoer, an easygoing guy, self-assured, and of course, a seducer who has never lacked women in his life again.

Of course, it wasn't an easy or quick journey. It took me time to get where I am now, but the first step was recognizing my problem and being open to a change of personality in my life, but without ceasing to be myself, and well, that's what I did.

So, please, don't be discouraged if it's hard for you or if you get frustrated during the process. It's completely normal; it happens to all of us. So, when that crosses your mind, just think that... the master wasn't made overnight; first and foremost, he was a student. That's how everything works in life; everything is a process. You can't expect to be a Jedi without first being a Padawan.

As a piece of advice, I'll tell you that something that helped me a lot in overcoming shyness was thinking about how absurd this problem was in itself. I thought about everything I was missing out on in this wonderful life simply because I didn't have the guts to face reality. Therefore, I committed myself to wanting to improve myself day by day, to gain confidence in myself, and ultimately, to leave the worst version of myself in the past.

If you've read this personal story carefully, you'll have noticed the keys to overcoming shyness. If you haven't, read it again until you identify the principles for overcoming it that are contained in this brief personal story. In any case, in the following chapters, you'll discover more keys to overcome it and to change your mindset to a successful one.

To conclude the chapter, I'll leave you with some small exercises to help you overcome shyness.

<u>Exercise</u>

1. **Identify the origin of your shyness**: Make a list of the situations or circumstances in which you feel the most shy. Try to identify the origin of your shyness. Was it caused by any particular event? Does it have to do with your self-image? Which type of shyness do you identify with the most? Once you've identified the origin, you can start working to overcome your shyness.

2. **Face your fears**: Think of a situation in which you feel particularly shy. Challenge yourself to face that situation. If you're afraid of public speaking, try speaking at a meeting or dinner with friends. If you're afraid of talking to a woman you like, approach her and start a conversation. With each small step you take, you'll feel more confident and less shy.

3. **Practice gradual exposure**: Gradual exposure is a technique that involves facing your fears gradually. If you're afraid of public speaking, for example, you can start by speaking in front of a small group of friends or family, then in a larger group, and finally in public. This

technique allows you to face your fears gradually, which will help you feel more comfortable and confident in situations that make you shy. Start by identifying a situation that makes you shy and establish a series of gradual steps that you can follow to face it.

4. **Step out of your comfort zone**: Do something you wouldn't normally do. If you're shy, you're likely to feel more comfortable doing the things you always do. Step out of your comfort zone and do something new, something that challenges you. It can be as simple as taking a dance class, a cooking workshop, or a group sport. From my perspective, what I always recommend and what is best, is to take a solo trip. With each new experience you have, you'll feel more confident, you'll be forced to interact with unfamiliar people, and it will therefore be easier for you to overcome that condition of shyness.

LET'S CHANGE MINDSETS!

CHAPTER II

In the previous chapter, we discussed shyness, its reasons, and how to overcome it. So if the reading has been clear... I suppose you'll understand that a change of mindset is needed to overcome this barrier and inconvenience, which prevents you from moving forward in your normal, romantic, professional, and any other life aspect. Unfortunately, I can't change your mindset by magic or African witchcraft; it's a job you have to do yourself, and it solely depends on you. But I can give you a series of guidelines and advice to help unlock your mind and become the seducer you desire.

But, before we get into that, let me tell you another personal story because I firmly believe that you'll learn more from real, lived anecdotes than from a bunch of cheap and unreadable theory that only makes you want to throw the book out the window. Let's start with the story.

It was the year 2016. At that time, I was living in London, twenty years old, and working as a bartender at a Mexican bar in Stratford called Wahaca. As usual, I had a coworker I liked, whom I found very attractive. However, as I've told you before, I was still shy and found it hard to interact. Nevertheless, I was aware of my problem and wanted to change it at all costs. So one day, after a long time and almost stuttering, I decided to take action. I asked her out for a drink after work, to which she agreed.

The date itself was quite normal; we went for a drink, talked, and talked even more. But nothing serious happened, not even a kiss, so we each went home to sleep, alone in our beds. We continued to meet after work about four more times, going for walks, to the movies, for meals, and other things people usually do on a date.

It was clear that she liked me, but I simply didn't have the guts to tell her. My shyness, coupled with the fear of rejection, paralyzed me and prevented me from acting naturally and confidently. As you can see, I was my own enemy, sabotaging myself with self-inflicted insecurities, without any logic or reason.

The breaking point came when I invited her to my house for dinner. I asked my roommate to leave so I could have the place to myself, as I was sharing a room and a house with nine other people at that time. (Rent in London was expensive, and I had no choice but to live that way.)

The conclusion is that we ended up in my bed watching a movie. Hours passed, and I didn't make a move; I didn't even dare to kiss her. Negative thoughts raced through my head—I told myself that she might reject me if I made a move, or worse, she might get angry and leave. To add more fuel to the fire, we worked together, so I told myself that she might speak ill of me to my colleagues, and then they would look at me differently at work and laugh at me. In short, lots of mental dramas and absurd paranoia worthy of a bad horror movie.

Luckily, all of that was just in my head; it was science fiction and didn't happen in the real world. So, I pushed aside all those negative and toxic thoughts, made a mental effort to overcome them, and finally mustered the courage to kiss her. To my surprise, she eagerly returned the kiss, and we ended up spending the night together. In case you're curious, we continued to see each other for a while until I left London.

The funny thing about all of this is that when I kissed her for the first time, she jokingly said she thought I would never do it, that she had the impression that I didn't like her and only wanted to be her friend, which was not my intention at all. But because of my cowardice and shyness, I gave that impression. The reason? Not having enough confidence in myself to express how I felt.

Imagine what would have happened if I hadn't decided to take action. I can assure you that if I hadn't acted that night, it's highly likely that I would have ended up in the friend zone, as she would have grown tired of me no matter how much she liked me. Besides, she would have seen me as a man who didn't have enough confidence to express his thoughts, so I would have lost all attractiveness immediately. It's well known that as a general rule, women get tired of men who don't take the initiative.

As you can see if you've paid attention to the story, most of the time, we are our own worst enemy. We invent things that will never happen out of simple imaginary fears, and we don't act because we let ourselves be carried away by our thoughts and the toxic ideas that torment us.

This often happens because we program ourselves with a negative mindset. You know what all the personal development gurus say: "Tell yourself you're going to be poor, and you will be." "Tell yourself you're going to be rich, and you'll have a high chance of becoming so." "Tell yourself you're ugly, and everyone will see you as such." "Tell yourself you're confident, and everyone will see you as confident." I could go on with plenty of examples, but I imagine you get the idea.

As you can see, the words we use and the way we talk to ourselves influence the actions we take or the ones we let pass because of those same thoughts, whether they are positive or negative.

So, what you have to ask yourself now is what kind of mindset you want. Do you want to continue being a victim of the system and of yourself? Do you want to stick with that toxic and negative mindset that won't bring you anything in life? Or, on the contrary, would you like to develop a positive mindset of success and abundance?

I imagine you've already chosen the path of success, abundance, and the courage to always move forward. Great! You've just taken the first step to becoming the next Mister Casanova. The master and owner of yourself. But first, my friend, POSITIVE AND SEDUCTIVE MINDSET!

Next, I'm going to propose a series of practical exercises to help you develop a positive mindset and reach your goal faster.

Exercise

1. **Focus on gratitude**. It sounds obvious and everyone says it, but it's very important because if you're a grateful person and you're aware, life will make more sense and you'll see things in a positive light. Make a list of reasons to be thankful for in life, it could be your family, your friends, your health, a house by the beach... it's up to you to do this exercise.

2. **Focus your attention on the present**. Don't worry too much about the past or the future. Instead, focus your attention on the present moment and the opportunities you have right now. This can help you feel more positive and focused. After all, as the Romans used to say, "CARPE DIEM".

3. **Surround yourself with positive people**. I'm sure you know people who always have a positive attitude, start hanging out with them and try to absorb their energy. Avoid negative, toxic, and insecure people as they will also transmit their negative energy to you.

4. **Be clear about your strengths and be proud of them**. Make a list of your skills

and positive characteristics as an individual. For example, you can be funny, intelligent, play a musical instrument, be good at a sport, and many more...

5. **Set realistic goals**. Write down your short-term goals in seduction and personal development, and even if you're thinking about starting a business, it would be good to write it down too.

6. **Visualize yourself as a winner and successful**. Think about everything you want to be, how you want to be, and constantly visualize it when you feel stuck, think about this and it will help you move forward.

Take this seriously because if you don't have the right mindset, you'll never become the seducer you want to be, it's the first step and you can't skip it.

If you haven't read my book *"Seductive Mindset: How to Flirt with Women"* yet, I recommend it, as I focus more on changing the mindset from negative to seductive and, of course, many other topics that I don't cover in this book. You can find it in the same store where you purchased this book if you're interested or feel like helping me continue with this project. If you're not interested, move on to the next chapter, from my side, I'm still happy to share this knowledge with you.

DO YOU WANT TO BE A WOLF OR A LAMB?

CHAPTER III

Unfortunately, and at the same time fortunately, life is full of slaughtered lambs, victims, purposeless individuals, followers of the masses, and those without life goals. It's the reason why the world functions as it does, with bosses and slaves, the poor and the rich, successful people and those who are not, those who succeed in dating and those who do not. It's the expression of life itself, it's natural, and it has always been and will continue to be so.

The fortunate aspect of this is that since lambs abound in the world, being a wolf makes you stand out above the rest and gain more value in the eyes of any individual. In fact, if you read any biographies of important people, they were self-made individuals, forged in fire and flame, solitary when they needed to be, and as cunning as wolves to seize the opportunities that life presented them.

Historical figures such as Hannibal, Napoleon, Hadrian, Marco Polo, and a long list of others were wolves, and most likely great seducers, as they didn't care about the opinion of others and did what they believed was best in every moment. Even if they made mistakes sometimes, the important thing is that they made decisions and acted upon them, without taking into account the opinion of the sheep. They were leaders and acted as such, causing admiration or respect from the rest of the individuals.

Relating this to seduction, you may have noticed that women don't like insecure men, purposeless men, or "little lambs". Unless... what they want is to dominate you, then they do like that. So unless you want to be dominated, in which case I would recommend a book on female domination. (I want to think that's not your case, and that you're still interested in reading this book).

So I understand that what you want is to be a Damn Wolf! Hungry for success, self-improvement, and women. So I invite you to go out and hunt for whatever you desire in life. Because while the lamb is fed, the wolf has to find its own food, and when it needs to, it eats the occasional lamb. This may sound cruel, but that's life, and it's in our hands to choose what kind of personality we want to be.

And you might be wondering... "Well... what does this have to do with seduction?" The answer is everything, plain and simple. To be a seducer, you have to become a wolf. The wolf adapts to its environment, it can go in a pack or alone, it can make long marches through any terrain, with an empty stomach, seeking the next prey to eat, without crying, without lamenting, knowing that it will find something, always surpassing itself. At the same time, it can strategize with its peers to obtain its food and ensure its survival. The wolf doesn't settle and always wants more, whether as a lone wolf or for its pack, but it always seeks a way, no matter how difficult, to survive.

This, my friend, translated to the human being, means being yourself, without caring a damn what others think, bringing out your own personality, going all out for your goals and purposes, making a living differently from the rest, breaking from convention, being authentic, remaining unfazed by criticism, overcoming rejection without caring, inviting the girl you like to dance at the club, or speaking fearlessly to the one you're interested in on the street or at work, expressing your ideas without hesitation, and above all, bringing out your best version.

Undoubtedly, like the wolf, everything I mentioned above are the characteristics of a seducer. That's why it's our duty as individuals to work on what we believe is convenient in each moment and what's best for each occasion. If your goal today is to become a seducer, capable of talking to the girl you like and taking her to bed, capable of being alone, capable of being in company when you feel like it, capable of being a person who is liked and attracts women because of their personality. If you want all of this... you must act like a wolf and acquire that mentality. Because this world is already full of sheep, and to be liked, stand out, or seduce, you need to offer something different, something new, while conveying calmness, naturalness, and confidence. All of these are keys to being a seducer.

So, wolf attitude, buddy, wolf attitude! I hope this has motivated you to change your mindset from "shy to seducer" or following this analogy, from "sheep to wolf." Let's reinforce what we've learned with a story of how I stopped being a little lamb and started to show the ears of the wolf. Before going to London, as I've already told you, I was a pretty shy and insecure guy, but I always had the internal spark to want to do things differently from the rest.

At that time, I was twenty years old. I had been working for a year in a meat factory, so I had some money saved up. I decided to take a solo trip around Europe to gain confidence and because I had never been out of Spain before, and I was curious to see more of the world.

The decision wasn't easy because I was a bit scared to travel alone, but I gathered my courage and decided to start the journey. I began in Italy, where I spent the first few days alone. Despite staying in a hostel, I found it quite challenging to interact with unknown people due to my shyness. So, I dedicated myself to solo sightseeing, which was fine, but I missed human company a bit. On the third day, luckily, some guys approached me and suggested going out to explore Rome together. I gathered my courage and decided to spend a few days with them while sightseeing, eating pizza, and having some Peroni. In this situation, I was forced to overcome my shyness and talk to strangers.

This helped me a lot in overcoming my fear of interacting with people I didn't know at all. Obviously, I still had my issues in my head, but let's say it was the first step towards change. It opened my eyes to socializing because, for me, it was a huge effort to start hanging out with people I didn't know at all. But at the same time, it was very rewarding and necessary for my mindset change.

My next destination was Denmark. As soon as I arrived at the hostel in the evening, I went to have a beer alone on the terrace. I imagine I must have seemed a bit pitiful to the others; I think they could tell I was an insecure and inexperienced young man. So, a group of locals there invited me to go out partying with them, to which I accepted without hesitation.

They were very friendly to me, introduced me to their friends, and even said that if I liked any of the girls, they wouldn't have any problem introducing me to them. I said yes, I gathered my courage, and I talked a bit with the girls. The reality is that I wasn't confident enough to take the first step, let alone end up in bed with one of them. So, it remained only as a somewhat basic conversation because I didn't have the necessary social skills to have a good conversation and seduce a woman. However, I continued to improve my social skills.

I'm sure I caught the attention of that girl because she showed interest in me. But in my head, the typical excuses of "how could she like me if...," or "she probably doesn't find me attractive because..." and a thousand others were still going through my mind.

Days went by, I met more people, had a great time, but I still couldn't control my emotions and my internal game. I was still a young Padawan when it came to seduction and social skills, but I was learning little by little without getting frustrated. Persistent as an ant, I was overcoming my shyness.

I left Denmark to visit a friend who was on Erasmus in Poland, specifically in Krakow, so I stayed at his place for a few days. The truth is, even though

I still couldn't manage to hook up (I was a complete loser), at least my social skills had improved considerably. I felt looser and more free to talk to people. In short, I wasn't as afraid of talking to strangers anymore, so I was leaving my shyness behind. (As you can see, it was all about consistency and practice.)

In Poland, I met a lot of people. There was a girl I really liked. She would come to talk to me, but I must confess that I still felt a lot of embarrassment when interacting with women. I got quite flustered and would turn red with a simple "hello". This, coupled with my poor English at the time, made the conversation difficult. Moreover, I still had blocks and didn't know how to advance the conversation, let alone how to seduce her. The science of seduction was still slipping through my fingers.

My stay in Krakow was filled with parties, feasting, a bit of sightseeing, and quite a few wanks, unfortunately. After that, I decided that I had to learn English if I wanted to maintain that lifestyle, so I decided to move to London to live, to learn it, and to put myself to the test even more. Luckily, I was quite aware that I needed to overcome myself to change my mindset from shy to seductive.

Before leaving, I passed through Prague. Undoubtedly a beautiful medieval city. There, I met some very cute Korean girls with whom I had some really good moments. To this day, I still regret not having had the balls to take action and do something more with them because in the end, I've always been left wondering what would have happened if I had taken action... I'll never know. Nevertheless, I still cherish a beautiful memory, and those negative experiences have taught me and made me the man I am now. As you can see, everything takes a process. (I won't tire of saying it until it's engraved in your subconscious).

The last stage of my trip was spent in Berlin, where I met more people and more women, but without success in terms of dating. (Yes, I was still killing myself with masturbation). I went out partying, visited all the important museums in the city, ate many Bratwursts, and drank some good German beers. Finally, after a few days, I went to London, where as I said, I decided to go to learn English, but that's another story that I have told a little earlier.

The conclusion of this story is that even though I hadn't hooked up with anyone during the whole trip, I hadn't even gotten a simple kiss, at least it gave me enough courage to start believing in myself. Traveling alone helped me discover that I was capable of developing social skills, so it helped me a lot to reinforce my inner confidence and self-assurance. Additionally, it helped me a lot to put my shyness aside a little more. In the end, traveling alone meant that I had to fend for myself without depending on anyone, only myself. So, I learned a lot about myself and saw what I was capable of.

It is true that I was still a little lamb, and I was still far from becoming the wolf that I am now, but I took the first step towards changing my mindset and attitude. It would still take a couple more years for me to become a wolf, so if you feel that you still don't have enough courage or confidence, don't get frustrated, this is a journey and it takes step by step, you can't reach the top without climbing the mountain first. Patience, good handwriting, and... Start changing your limiting mindset today! I'm sure you won't regret it.

<u>Exercise</u>

If you want to have the mindset of a seducer or a wolf, I'm going to give you a series of activities that I want you to do no matter what, without the option to reject or postpone them, and start doing them as quickly as possible.

1. **Go out partying alone**. It may seem like a big challenge or even loser-ish, but quite the opposite, this way you'll see what you're made of, you'll test yourself, and most likely discover qualities and capabilities you didn't know you had. The more times you do it, the better, it's not enough to do it just once. Commit to going out alone at least once every two weeks. Please, interact with women, it will be useless to stay silent and lonely all night. The goal here is to talk and interact, and if you can, end up with her that same night. It will probably go wrong the first few times, but... I dare you! (Personally, I hook up more when I go out alone than when I'm in bad company).

2. **Take a solo trip**. This is very much related to what I was saying in the previous exercise, but with the difference that by doing it, you'll grow much more as a person, you'll get to know yourself

better, and you'll forge a great personality as well as mindset. In fact, one of
the best things that happened to me in
life is traveling solo around the world,
I've spent 6 months in Southeast Asia,
traveled around North Africa, toured
Europe, and lived alone in London and
Switzerland. All of this solo, of course,
and I can tell you that I've always had
company when I felt like it and when
I wasn't, I was alone. I'll tell you some
stories later for sure. So do yourself a
favor and take a solo trip. You don't
have to be as crazy as me and go to the
other side of the world solo and without a defined time, but you can start by
going to the city next to where you live
and spend a weekend there to see how
it goes. I'm sure it will be very beneficial
for you to forge a wolf mindset.

3. **Talk to the girl you like already**. I don't
give a shit about the fear it gives you,
and the 159 mental excuses you come up
with, seriously, I don't care. Do it now!
Greet her and invite her out, for dinner, drinks, or whatever you feel like, but
you're already picking up your phone
and texting her on WhatsApp, Instagram, or whatever she uses. In the end,
you have nothing to lose and a lot to gain

because if she says yes, it's crazy, and if she says no, then you get rid of a weight off your shoulders because you know she's not interested, so you can focus on others. Come on, write to her! Are you a Lamb or a wolf?

The only exercise you have to do now is number three, that's indisputable. You'll do number one this coming weekend, with the goal of at least talking to a stranger woman that night. Number two, if you have money, you'll do it the following weekend, and if not, save up and do it as soon as possible. It's very important that you do them all, I assure you it will be much easier for you to change the mindset of a lamb and become a wolf, a seducer, a man confident in himself who knows what he wants. Have some balls! (If you think it's still too early and you don't feel ready, I can understand, but by the end of the book, you have to do them without excuses.)

Go for it, Wolf!

THE POWER OF BEING YOURSELF

CHAPTER IV

Have you ever seen a wolf wearing a mask? I'm sure you haven't. Continuing with the metaphor from the previous chapter, you'll agree with me that the wolf acts in a natural, innate way, learned to be as it is because of the hostile nature, and also from its wolf mother who taught it how to survive. It's true that there are stronger and weaker wolves, just like there are Alphas of the pack, but in the end, they are all wolves and each one has a special quality that makes them stand out one way or another from the rest.

Given all this information, you will have realized that the wolf acts by nature and does not pretend to be someone it's not. On the contrary, humans tend to act behind false masks like those of a Venetian carnival. Simply due to lack of self-love, a lack of an exciting life, or rather, out of fear of showing who they really are, and even because they don't know who they really are. Acting in this way, behind masks, without showing your true personality, will distance you from being a seducer, and will bring you closer to being a counterfeit piece of Chinese clothing. That's why it's very important to be yourself, to know yourself, and not to pretend to be someone you're not. If you still don't know who you are, you have another task to add to your to-do list.

I'm not saying this, but rather the famous oracle of Delphi, with its famous "Know yourself." Therefore, if you want to be a seducer, the first thing you must do is to know yourself and BE YOURSELF. Ask yourself, search for what you like and are passionate about. Who are you? Where do you want to go? What are you good at? What are you bad at? What are your ambitions or purposes? Where do you see yourself in 5 years? What is your purpose for reading this book? Search for your natural essence, and reflect on this.

As the wolf you have decided to be, you must be very clear about the importance of naturalness when seducing women. It's time to unleash the wolf within you and bring out your true self! You have to recognize that there is no one like you and therefore feel special, unique, and try to bring out your best version.

Showing yourself as you are, confident and fearless, will convey a lot of security and confidence in an indirect way. This is something women love, as they value it very positively, so they will be much more receptive to giving you a chance to get to know you.

What would you prefer if you were a woman? To go out with someone who pretends to be something they're not, and uses copy-and-paste techniques they learned from a seduction guru? Or, to go out with someone who knows what they want, who is authentic and confident in themselves?

So, if you've chosen the correct answer, I would like to invite you to forget all those cheap seduction techniques you may have learned from other gurus or books, as they are just copy-and-paste that won't work for you. These techniques don't adapt to all types of personalities, which will make you sound forced or ridiculous. Believe me when I say that women notice this right away. Avoid making a fool of yourself and start being original!

In this world of copies, you must be the best version of yourself in order to stand out, to be with many more women, if that's what you want, and for any other aspect of your personal life.

But Giovanni, all this is great, but... How do I do it? How do I become more authentic, be myself?

Unfortunately, I can't give you an exact answer, as each person is a different world, so it's up to you to roll up your sleeves and get to work. To be authentic, it is essential that you take the time to explore who you really are, what you are passionate about, what your values are, and what sets you apart from others. Reflect on your life experiences, your achievements, your challenges, and how they have shaped you up to this point.

Once you have a deeper understanding of yourself, you must embrace your true personality and show it to the world. Don't worry about pleasing others or fitting into a pre-established mold. Instead, focus on being true to your own beliefs, values, and principles.

Remember that being authentic doesn't mean being perfect. Don't be afraid to show your weaknesses, as they are part of life, but also make sure to showcase your strengths and share your experiences. Women love honest and sincere men, as it is true that they connect more with those who show themselves just as they are, as God brought them into the world. (I'm not referring to nudity, which they also like, but that's not the case now).

To become yourself, you must believe in your abilities, in your qualities, and in your capacity to attract women. Confidence and authenticity are two very attractive characteristics, which draw people, or in this case, women, towards you. Work on strengthening your self-esteem and recognizing your own worth.

Finally, remember that being authentic is a continuous process. Allow yourself to grow, evolve, and explore new facets of your personality. Authenticity isn't about stagnating in a static version of yourself but about allowing yourself to be who you really are at every moment of your life. You won't be the same today as you will be in twenty years, so continuing to grow as a person should be a lifestyle for you.

I'll give you an example of what not to do if you want to be a true seducer. I have a friend whom we'll call David. David is a guy who looks good, is attractive, and is fun.

The problem with David is that he doesn't feel good about himself, doesn't accept who he is, and doesn't accept the circumstances that have happened in his life. He recently divorced his wife, with whom he has a daughter. Obviously, it's a traumatic experience, and my friend went through a rough time. He quit his job, moved back in with his mother, and was practically broke. In short, he was screwed.

Instead of facing his problem and trying to find a solution, being himself to move forward with his flaws and virtues, David decided, on the contrary, to invent a fictional character. A personality that wasn't his own, to avoid his problems and try to attract other women, as in the end, that's what he was seeking, to alleviate his sorrows with another woman, even if it was only sexually.

With this fictional character, I found myself one day at a bar. I was trying to cheer him up because he's my friend, and I felt really bad that he was going through a rough patch. So, I get up, introduce myself to a group of women, and they let us sit with them. So far, so good; we were having the typical conversation you have when you meet someone new. "Where are you from? What are you doing around here? What do you like to do? What are your names?" and all that...

As usual, one of the girls asked my friend David what he did for a living, to which he said he had a car buying and selling business, and that he not only sold in Spain but throughout Europe, that he made a lot of money, had a very busy life, and ultimately, that he was the best thing since sliced bread.

David was stiffer than a board; he had no money at all, and it was I who was inviting him out at that moment. My friend's luck was that, in the end, he was likable to women; they laughed with him, and ultimately, he managed to pick up girls. The problem was that eventually, the lies would collapse under their own weight because, besides, he used to say he had a car when his car was repossessed due to debts.

David would meet the girl again, and of course,

the lies couldn't be sustained anymore. They realized he had no money, no company, his car never showed up to pick them up, and ultimately, David was a liar. This doesn't attract women; on the contrary, it repels them. It might work for a one-night stand, especially if you have a friend like me who pays the expenses. But generally, he couldn't even get laid because, in the end, women's characteristic sixth sense would expose him before he even got them into bed.

My friend ended up in a pretty bad state, as he invented a character and didn't face his problems. He fell into drugs, bad company, and was dishonest with everyone. He told fictitious stories to take advantage of people, both men and women. Maybe he succeeded sometimes, but in the end, he ended up alone, and he's currently in a rehab. I hope that at least, learning from his mistakes, and trying to be himself again. I don't have contact with him at the moment, but I hope everything goes well for him, and he can come out of this better than before.

So please, don't be like my friend David; as much as I care about him, his decisions to pretend to be someone he wasn't made him end up very badly. That's why it's so important to be oneself at all times, with honesty, values, and respect. I assure you that's what attracts women the most. By being yourself, you'll not only get laid one day, but if you do it right, you can be with whoever you want, for as long as you want, have sex as many times as you want, or have a healthy relationship, depending on what you're looking for.

In conclusion and to close this chapter, there's no magic formula, but the path to authenticity begins with self-exploration, confidence in yourself, honest communication with yourself and those around you, and constant personal growth. Follow this path, and you'll see how you become an authentic and attractive man, capable of seducing from your true self. Trust yourself! Be authentic! And become a wolf!

Now, I invite you to do the following exercise that will help you get to know yourself better while bringing out your best version. It's essential to take the necessary time and energy to do it; otherwise, it won't be productive.

<u>Exercise</u>

1. **Acknowledge your passions and life purposes**. Make a list of things that you are passionate about, as well as your life goals or what you want to achieve in the short and medium term, and try to apply them to your daily life. This will help you connect with your inner self and bring out your authenticity as an individual. - For example, if you enjoy traveling, then travel more often. If your goal is to be a seducer and flirt with more women, write it down and think about what characteristics you need to achieve it.

2. **Define your seductive personality**. Reflect and write about your own personality and relate it to seduction. What kind of seducer would you like to be? How would you like your relationships with women to be? Therefore, see yourself as a seducer already and write down what qualities, characteristics, and seductive behaviors you would have. When you do this, put that role in sight to reinforce your idea of who you want to be, and in this way, force yourself to acquire those personal development qualities you lack and want to become.

3. **Analyze your fears, what prevents you from becoming the seducer you want to be**. Make a list of your fears and limitations regarding seduction, interactions with women, and personal development. Reflect on how these fears have held you back and prevent you from being who you want to be. Then, write down specific strategies to overcome each fear and limitation, focusing on how you can face them and grow personally.

4. **The mirror technique**. It may sound like complete nonsense, but it is a very effective and not so well-known technique to boost self-confidence and achieve the goals you set for yourself. The technique consists of looking at yourself in a mirror in the eyes and telling yourself the positive characteristics that you have, as well as what you will achieve in life. - For example, tell yourself how confident and attractive you are, how capable you are of getting the woman you set your sights on, so you are worth it and you know it, reaffirm it, speak to yourself positively and believe it. Try to do this at least once a day for about 5 to 10 minutes in a space where you feel comfortable.

5. **Memorize the following principles you have learned in this reading**.

- **Adopt the mindset of the wolf**: Abandon the mindset of the lamb and assume a strong and independent mentality. Trust in your own worth and pursue your goals with determination.

- **Overcome shyness and build social skills**: Face your fears and develop your verbal and non-verbal communication skills. Learn to initiate and maintain interesting conversations.

- **Be authentic and discover your seductive personality**: Recognize that each person is unique and has their own seductive personality. Discover your passions and life purpose, define your seductive personality, and face your fears and limitations.

- **Cultivate self-confidence**: Work on your self-esteem, visualize yourself as a successful seducer, and use positive language to strengthen your mindset. Believe in yourself and your abilities.

- **Reinforce your authenticity through the mirror exercise**: Look at your reflection honestly and recognize your qualities. Affirm yourself in your worth and commit to being authentic in your interactions with women.

It is very important that you do not proceed with the reading until you have completed these exercises. I know you would love to continue reading, but self-control yourself, take the necessary time to complete these exercises, concentrate, and do your best.

¡LIVE A UNIQUE LIFE!

CHAPTER V

As a Wolf and the man you've chosen to be, leading a unique, fulfilling, and envy-inducing life is another hallmark of a seducer. You'll know that most people lead dull, monotonous, emotionless, and meaningless lives, so they'll never catch anyone's attention because they follow lives that everyone hates and does.

Generally, these kinds of people play in the rat race, always being poor or slaves to a job or boss, with no control over their time, little room for personal development, and entirely dependent on a life they can't escape from but constantly complain about.

"But Guatson? What does this have to do with seduction?"

Well... simply put, nobody is attracted to a monotonous life. If your goal is to seduce women, having a systematic life in which you don't control your time makes things complicated. I'm not saying it's impossible, but it's easier to attract someone if you lead a different, fulfilling life full of emotions and financial freedom because the different always attracts more, and this is an undeniable fact. Because here's a secret: most of the women you're attracted to are longing to meet someone who can pull them out of their routine, boring, and meaningless life. So, if you're a dull guy without purpose and trapped in monotony, it'll be harder for you to pull that woman out of her routine because you don't even know how to get out of your own.

Who would you prefer to meet? A waitress who only goes from work to home? or A woman who is entrepreneurial, a traveler, and in control of her time?

The woman you're trying to flirt with would have chosen the same answer.

Don't get me wrong; I'm not telling you to quit your job right now and leave behind your monotonous and boring life. I imagine you have fixed expenses like everyone else, which need to be paid. Quitting your job or studies right now isn't the smartest idea. However, what I'm trying to say is that you should start acquiring knowledge about other areas, such as financial freedom or business, so you can aspire to have that different life and get to work on it as soon as you can.

On the other hand, you don't need to be rich to travel, experience other cultures, and ultimately do whatever you damn well please, but money certainly helps, especially in the global system we live in. Therefore, it will help you build a different life. So, keep doing what you're doing so far, but focus on aspiring to something more, be different, and try to lead a different life. You can be a hippie living in a caravan; that would also make you different and there's nothing wrong with that. But from my point of view, I prefer to start a business, write a book, have an email marketing list that generates online income, and allows me to live the lifestyle I like, which would also enable me to live in a caravan if I desire. (Which I consider doing someday).

Let me give you an example to make it clear, Philip II, the father of Alexander the Great, is a clear example of someone who stood out from the rest and led an extraordinary life.

This man was the youngest son of a Macedonian king, so inheriting the throne was almost impossible for him. To add more difficulty, he was sent as a hostage to the neighboring kingdom of Thebes due to a military defeat of his father against this same kingdom, which could have resulted in him never returning home. However, after returning to Macedonia, facing off against his brothers, the support of some military personnel, and a bit of luck, he managed to inherit the throne.

Not content with that, he was also the creator of the famous Macedonian Phalanx and, to top it off, put Macedonia on the map of ancient Greece with his successful military campaigns when it was once nothing more than a kingdom in decline. Creating the Corinthian League, he became the greatest power and reference point for the entire Peloponnesian region at that time.

He didn't stop there; he was also well-known for boosting the morale of his troops, as he liked to fight on foot and on the front lines of battle (when all the nobles of the time went on horseback), earning not only the respect of all the kingdoms he conquered but also of his own soldiers and comrades. In doing so, he lost an eye and was wounded in a leg, which left him limping for life.

On a sentimental level, he had 7 wives and only God knows how many more mistresses, all attracted to him by his power and extraordinary life. (Unfortunately, it is said that the last woman had him assassinated out of jealousy) So you can get an idea of how many women he was with.

It was also thanks to him that Alexander the Great could lead another life of envy, as he left him an empire on the rise and a new army, reformed and the best of the time, which took him all the way to India.

Even today, almost three thousand years later,

his feats and exploits are still recounted as an example of someone who decided to surpass himself, achieve accomplishments that no one had ever reached or even dreamed of before, and forever mark ancient history. All this for deciding to lead an extraordinary life and not settle for the secondary role of being the younger son.

Granted, what I'm telling you happened many years ago, and well, he was also the son of a king, but the idea is for you to grasp his extraordinary life and everything he did. Which made him enviable in the eyes of other men, and irresistible in the eyes of any woman. Best of all, both men and women would feel the same even in modern times.

With this, you don't have to be a Macedonian king to lead a successful and fulfilling life, but you do need to understand the difference between living a life of abundance and success, or living a life of submission, normalcy, and anonymity.

This chapter is just a piece of advice, to be engraved in your subconscious, as it's not the most relevant when it comes to seducing a woman, but it is something that will make a huge difference and facilitate the task much more, simply due to the admiration you can cause in the other person. Simply for being a self-made man, who achieves his goals, objectives, leads a dream life, is financially independent, and couldn't care less what others think, because he knows what he wants and how to get it.

As a wolf and seducer that you want to be, this should be one of your life goals, not only to flirt and meet women, but for yourself, to lead a fulfilling life, of which you feel proud to tell your peers, friends, flings, your future wife, or your grandchildren.

Well, I'm going to go have a beer, and prepare for my trip to Mallorca, where I'm going tomorrow with a beautiful woman I'm getting to know, to spend three days of beach, sun, good company, food, and great sex.

I might tell you how it goes in the next chapters, or I might decide to keep the story to myself, we'll see.

I'll leave you with a practical exercise so you can look for a business idea or an entrepreneurial venture so you too can lead a different life if you feel like it.

<u>Exercise</u>

1: Discover Your Passions and Skills.

-Make a list of what you're passionate about and your key skills.

-Find the intersection between your passions and skills.

2: Identify Market Opportunities.

-Choose at least three areas of interest from the previous list.

-Research the market in each area to identify opportunities.

-Select the option that combines your interest with a market opportunity.

3: Define Your Unique Value Proposition.

-Describe how your project will address the market's needs or desires.

-Clearly define what sets you apart from the competition.

4: Develop an Action Plan.

-Set clear goals for your venture in the short, medium, and long term.

-Create a detailed action plan with concrete steps and deadlines.

5: Unlock Your First Entrepreneurial Move.

-Review your action plan and find the most accessible step to start.

-Is it sending emails to potential collaborators? Designing your project's logo? Researching suppliers? Buying a domain name? Writing a book?

-Execute this first step today, no matter how modest it may be.

ALPHA, BETA, SIGMA MALE

WHICH ONE DO YOU WANT TO BE?

CHAPTER VI

In this chapter, I wanted to discuss the differences between being an Alpha, a Beta, and a Sigma male, so that you can understand the characteristics of each one clearly, and so that you can choose which one you identify with the most in general terms, with the idea that this motivates you to make the change you are seeking in your life. Below, I explain each type of male profile in the field of seduction.

Alpha Male

Seductive Characteristics:

The Alpha male exudes unwavering confidence that naturally attracts female attention. His body language speaks of authority and power, with a penetrating gaze that communicates desire and determination. His self-assurance translates into a firm voice and assured gestures.

Relationship with Seduction:

The Alpha, in the realm of seduction, is characterized by taking the initiative naturally. He is not afraid to express his intentions clearly, creating a dynamic where the woman feels desired and guided. His ability to lead in seduction lies in the combination of confidence, humor, and an instinctive understanding of female desires.

Perception by Women:

From a woman's perspective, the Alpha Male represents the fantasy of a strong and self-assured man. The Alpha's security and determination generate a visceral attraction, while his ability to lead in seduction creates an exciting and passionate atmosphere.

Advantages:

- Immediate attraction.
- Dynamism and natural leadership.

- Excitement and passion in the relationship.

<u>Disadvantages:</u>

- May be perceived as arrogant.
- Possible lack of deep emotional connection.
- High expectations that can create pressure.

Beta Male:

Seductive Characteristics:

The Beta Male stands out for his empathy and ability to emotionally connect. In the game of seduction, his charm lies in his ability to understand the desires and needs of the woman, creating a genuine connection. His relaxed and friendly attitude contributes to a comfortable and welcoming atmosphere.

Relationship with Seduction:

Unlike the Alpha, the Beta approaches seduction from an emotional connection. He excels at listening attentively, showing genuine interest, and expressing his own emotions. His focus is on building a relationship beyond the superficial, creating a connection based on authenticity and mutual understanding.

Perception by Women:

For women, the Beta Male represents emotional security and meaningful connection. The Beta's ability to understand and support creates an atmosphere of trust and closeness. His charm lies in his authenticity and in creating a relationship based on mutual understanding.

Advantages:

- Deep emotional connection.

- Relaxed and comfortable atmosphere.
- Focus on communication and understanding.

Disadvantages:

- May be perceived as lacking leadership.
- Less initially attractive.
- High risk of being relegated to the "friendzone".

Sigma Male:

Seductive Characteristics:

The Sigma Male envelops himself in an air of mystery that is intriguing to women. His independence and reserved focus create an attraction based on curiosity. His body language suggests self-confidence, but in a more subtle and enigmatic way.

Relationship with Seduction:

In the game of seduction, the Sigma stands out for his less conventional approach. He does not follow traditional rules and prefers a more relaxed approach. His ability to maintain a certain degree of distance creates an intriguing dynamic where the woman is drawn to discovering more about him.

Perception by Women:

From the woman's perspective, the Sigma Male represents challenge and intrigue. His mystery generates an appeal based on curiosity and adventure. Women perceive the Sigma as someone who follows his own path, creating a sense of unpredictability and excitement in the relationship.

Advantages:

- Attraction based on curiosity.
- Independence and autonomy.

- Less pressure on traditional expectations.

<u>Disadvantages:</u>

- Difficulty in establishing commitments.
- May be perceived as distant.
- Less predictable in terms of leadership.

Perfect, you've already got an idea of each type of profile, its advantages, and its disadvantages. The important thing here is to grasp the concept that nobody in this world fits exactly into one type of profile, as if they were a robot; on the contrary, all human beings are flexible, adaptable, and have the power to choose how we want to be, acquiring and internalizing characteristics and abilities that we would like to have.

So don't be a robot, just be aware of the general traits of each profile type, adapt what you like best to your personality, work to acquire the social role you desire. Simply be natural and be yourself, taking into account all the characteristics listed earlier in this chapter.

Remember, there is no ideal profile type. We can all be seductive regardless of our characteristics. Personally, I identify with characteristics of all three types of seductive profiles. So, I don't let any one of them define me specifically; instead, I take the best characteristics from each one, make them my own, and shine through my naturalness.

PART II:

Unlocking the Art of Seduction;
Traits and Talents
of a True Seductor.

MASTER YOUR LOOK AND SEDUCE THROUGH STYLE!

In this chapter, I'll take you on the fascinating journey of seduction through personal image. The way you present yourself to the world says a lot about you and has a significant impact on your ability to attract women. You'll learn to develop a unique style that reflects your seductive personality and helps you stand out from the crowd.

Listen, buddy, before you can seduce a woman with your unique personal style, you first need to know what cards you're playing with, meaning your own body.

Take a moment in front of the mirror and see what terrain you're navigating. Notice your strengths, your weaknesses, and areas for improvement. Don't fool yourself or play dumb because if you don't know yourself, how the hell do you expect someone else to know you?

Identify your strengths, those physical attributes that make you stand out. It could be your charming hair, your Jonny Bravo arms, or that Spartan champion posture you rock. These are your aces up your sleeve, and it's time to show them to the world. But, hey, also be aware of your weaknesses and work on them. Don't hide behind excuses, buddy. It's time to take action and improve!

Once you've assessed your terrain, it's time to implement your dressing strategy. Choose clothes that highlight your best physical features and disguise the areas that make you feel insecure. Don't worry, I'm not saying you should wear a costume or blindly follow the latest fashion trends. The key is to find a balance between showcasing your unique personality and looking impeccable.

Experiment with different styles and find out which one suits you best. You can opt for a more casual yet elegant look, or maybe you prefer something more sophisticated and daring. Remember, style isn't just about the clothes you wear, but also about how you feel when you wear them. Dare to be authentic, blaze your own trail, and leave your mark with every step you take.

on't forget to pay attention to the details. Clean shoes, a hairstyle that reflects your personality, a good perfume, and accessories that show your good taste are small details that can make a difference, like a nice watch, a necklace, a bracelet, or something that holds emotional significance for you. The important thing is that you also feel comfortable with your choices.

Don't be a lazy bum, dedicate time and effort to your appearance. Remember, the image you project is the first impression women will have of you, so make sure it's an impression that at least catches attention positively.

Details are what differentiate between being "okay," "good," and being "extraordinary." Make sure to pay attention to every aspect of your appearance. Take care of your hair, keep your beard in shape, and choose clothes that fit your body and personal style. But don't forget that true style lies in the simple details.

Add distinctive touches to your style, like unique accessories that tell a story about who you are, about that trip you took, or that gift from a family member you cherish. Remember that details convey intentions and show that you care about every aspect of your appearance. Make every detail count, and you'll see how your seductive image rises to a whole new level!

Express confidence through your style. Seduction starts from within and is reflected in your personal style. When you feel good about yourself, it shows in how you dress and how you move through the world. Self-confidence is incredibly attractive, and your style can be a powerful tool to project it.

Don't be afraid to experiment and step out of your comfort zone. Try new styles and find those that make you feel like the most confident man in the room. Remember, style isn't about blindly following fashion rules but about being true to yourself and showing the world the best version of you. Trust yourself and let your seductive style shine!

Dare to be unique. In a world full of copies and stereotypes, stand out like a true gem in the crowd. Seduction is about being authentic and different at all times. Don't be afraid to stand out and be unique. Your uniqueness is your greatest strength and the key to capturing women's attention.

Break the barriers of conventionality and dare to be different. Experiment with colors, textures, and patterns that make you feel confident and powerful. Remember, the world doesn't need more imitators; it needs more brave and unique individuals who dare to shine with their own essence.

Don't be like my friend John. He has a style that's too unique and original. It's true that he's not the most attractive guy in the world, but that's not all. He doesn't take care of his appearance either; he has long, unkempt hair that definitely doesn't look good, along with a beard that seems like he's just returned from spending time with Robinson Crusoe on a deserted island.

To top it off, he doesn't dress very well either. Sure, he wears comfortable clothes, but he also has his own style that doesn't match anything, which makes even the island monkeys not pay attention to him.

My friend doesn't care about his image at all, which is why we all thought he was still a virgin, unless he's resorted to paying for a prostitute (whose information I'm unaware of). But I know he's been depressed about it lately, yet he doesn't do anything to change.

On the contrary, he prides himself on being different, which he certainly is, and a lot. That's great, and it's what I advocate for throughout this book, but his case is extreme. If you want a woman to notice you, you at least have to dedicate a minimum effort to your appearance because it doesn't matter if you're a great guy, if you look like a sideshow attraction, you won't appeal to anyone, not even your mother.

To top off the story, the last straw came a few days ago when I met up with him to take a walk because he had to pick up an order from Decathlon.

He confessed to me that it was three T-shirts from the hunting section, all in the same green color. To add insult to injury, he told me he had two more identical ones at home. Apparently, my friend's goal is to look like Bart Simpson, but with an even uglier shirt and almost twenty years apart. It's true that my friend John has female friends, but they all categorize him in the "friend zone" due to his lack of personal care and image. No woman finds him attractive, so they see him as a man without a spine.

If your intention is not to die a virgin like my friend John, to repel female glances, and to become a professional pussy dryer, do yourself a favor, and dedicate a bit of care to your image. Do everything in your power to look good and attract the attention of women, or at least not repel them.

In this chapter, you've learned the importance of cultivating a seductive personal style, without being like my friend John. From discovering your unique style to paying attention to details, expressing confidence, and daring to be different, every aspect of your personal image contributes to your seduction abilities. Remember, your style is a powerful tool that can open doors or close them, and it can either pique women's interest or push them away.

Next, I'm going to give you a list of 7 possible scenarios for a date, along with a simple clothing tip to look good, elegant, and convey confidence. These are just examples to give you a practical idea of how to dress well to catch attention, but they are just that: suggestions. If you have a better idea with which you think you'll feel more comfortable, go ahead and implement it without any fear. My idea is simply that you don't end up like my friend John.

7 Possible Date Scenarios and What to Wear.

Smart Casual Outfit for a Restaurant Date.

- Trousers: Wear well-fitting dark jeans. Consider wearing a black or dark belt.
- Shirt: Put on a button-up shirt, such as a white or checkered shirt that you like.
- Shoes: Opt for simple sneakers or shoes that you wear on a daily basis and try to match them with the trousers or shirt.
- Accessory: Carry a classic watch or wear a bracelet or any accessory you like.

Coffee Date.

- Trousers: Dark or colored jeans of your choice.
- T-shirt: Simple T-shirt in a color you like.
- Shoes: Comfortable sneakers you already own.
- Accessory: If you wear one, a simple cap can add a casual touch.

Casual Outfit for a Stroll.

- Trousers: Dress pants or comfortable fabric trousers.
- Shirt: Well-fitting button-up shirt.
- Shoes: Loafers or comfortable shoes.
- Accessory: A simple bracelet can add an interesting detail.

<u>*Outfit for a Casual Date or Day Game.*</u>

- Trousers: Dark or colored jeans of your choice.
- T-shirt: Simple T-shirt in a color you like.
- Shoes: Comfortable sneakers you already own.
- Accessory: You can add a hat if you feel comfortable or any other personal item you like.

<u>*Party Outfit.*</u>

- Trousers: Well-fitting dark trousers.
- Shirt: V-neck or round-neck shirt in a simple color.
- Shoes: Comfortable matching shoes.
- Accessory: Add a discreet necklace or chain for a stylish touch.

<u>*Outdoor Summer Date.*</u>

- Trousers: Comfortable shorts.
- T-shirt: T-shirt with a simple design.
- Shoes: Comfortable sports shoes.
- Accessory: A sporty cap can be practical and attractive, or wear nothing on your head as you prefer.

<u>*Casual Winter Date.*</u>

- Trousers: Dark jeans or chinos.

- Shirt: Flannel shirt in winter tones.
- Sweater: Round-neck or V-neck sweater in a color you like.
- Coat: Long wool coat in dark tones.
- Shoes: Leather boots or sturdy ankle boots.

MASCULINE ENERGY: THE KEY TO BEING A SEDUCER

CHAPTER VIII

Unfortunately, as you may already know, dear reader, in today's politicized and indoctrinated society, masculine energy is not well-regarded. In fact, from my point of view, there is an attempt to feminize men, making them less independent, weaker, more insecure, and ultimately easier to control and manipulate.

I dare say that this is nothing more than a strategy to achieve the absolute control sought by the world's elites. A way to manipulate the population at their whim, and what better way than to create herds of weak, insecure, confused men who don't know who they are, where they come from, or where they are going. I believe, and it is my mere opinion, that this is a very easy way to have those individuals under their control, to consume, work, and do what the leaders want.

It seems like a current trend that men now have to be as feminine as possible, forget their masculinity, their energy, and become someone who doesn't know who they are. I constantly see brats on the street who fit all these characteristics. I also see how society controls them, and they go like lambs to the slaughterhouse without any clear direction. Defending any new absurd law about progressivism or woke culture, without their own ideas, just going along with the current decadent trend that I observe. It's just my opinion.

The important thing about this brief personal reflection is that if you want to be a true seducer, in control of yourself, confident, who knows where he's going and what he wants in life, you should stay away from these new trends and cultivate your masculine energy. By this, I don't mean that you should be a caveman who fights for everything, kills, and makes rough sounds like "Unga, Unga". But you shouldn't be a lost man either, lacking in energy, who only conveys sadness and nothing else. The key lies in finding the middle ground.

Since ultimately the importance in seduction is the energy you transmit, much more important than how your attire looks or any superficial thing. What makes the difference when it comes to seducing, or even closing a sale, is the energy you transmit, what you radiate, how you look, every step you take, and how you smile. But before we delve into theories, let's define what masculine energy is.

Masculine Energy: For many, masculine energy evokes images of bravery and physical strength, and while these qualities may be part of it, masculine energy is much more than that. It's about that internal determination that drives us to face challenges and pursue our goals with burning passion. It's the courage to be authentic, to embrace our truth, and live with integrity. It's the art of not giving up and pursuing a goal until achieving it, regardless of circumstances or environment. It's decisiveness, leadership, confidence, and naturalness.

Imagine the lion on the savanna: majestic, protective, and full of confidence in its dominion. That's masculine energy at its core. It propels us to be leaders, not only in the traditional sense but as leaders of our own lives. When we radiate this energy, we send a clear message of self-assertion, security, confidence, while also generating attraction through our determination.

And what are the characteristics of masculine energy? I'll tell you next.

- **Confidence**: Masculine energy is often associated with self-confidence and decisiveness.

- **Physical and Mental Strength**: Traditionally, masculinity has been linked to physical strength and mental resilience.

- **Determination and Ambition**: Masculine energy is often associated with the determination to achieve goals and ambition in professional and personal life.

- **Independence**: The ability to be independent and self-reliant is seen as a characteristic of masculine energy.

- **Responsibility**: Assuming responsibilities and taking care of oneself and others are attributes often associated with masculine energy.

- **Leadership**: Masculine energy has historically been linked to leadership and decision-making.

- **Balanced Emotional Expression**: Although there is the idea that masculine energy may be less emotionally expressive, balanced emotional expression that does not repress emotions is valued.

- **Courage**: Willingness to face challenges and take risks is often considered part of masculine energy.

- **Problem-Solving Skills**: Masculine energy is often associated with the ability to analyze and solve problems logically.

Pay attention to those men who always attract women's glances, I'm sure you know at least one. Do you think it's just because of their looks or their demeanor? Does it influence? Of course it does, but the key is the energy they emit. They project their masculine energy, their eagerness to act, their self-confidence, their passion for life. It's this energy that women notice and makes them catch the eye and attention because ultimately, energy is perceived whether it's positive or not, and women notice it a lot. They have a much more developed perception of energy than men.

Now, pay attention, I'm going to give you a practical example of this energy. Imagine you're at a nightclub and a girl looks at you directly in the eyes. You automatically have two options:

A) You look away, adopt a hunched posture, trying to go unnoticed. The woman notices it and nothing happens, the interaction is over, as you transmitted an energy of insecurity and little masculinity, repelling any possibility of a positive interaction.

B) On the other hand, in the second example, you decide to maintain eye contact, keep your posture, smile at her, wink, and approach her to talk. (Since the woman has caught your attention and you find her attractive). This way, you are transmitting an energy of security, confidence, and masculinity.

If you communicate this masculine energy I'm talking about, it creates a kind of magic where you don't need to say anything because the woman in question will feel your presence and your energy. She won't be able to overlook you because your gaze will convey confidence and desire.

Obviously, at some point, you'll have to speak and say something, but here the important thing is to grasp the concept of energy and what you're capable of transmitting with your energy or aura. I'll address the topic of verbal and non-verbal communication in another chapter later on; for now, let's focus on masculine energy.

You must understand that confidence and security are key principles of seduction, and these are encompassed within the same masculine energy if you know how to channel it. I emphasize that when you act on your own steps, have your own goals, and are sure of yourself, women are attracted like a drunk to a bar. It's as if you assure them, without words, that they can feel comfortable and protected by your side. (I may be exaggerating a bit, but nevertheless, this is quite true as a general rule.)

You have to be clear that confidence doesn't come from arrogance but from a deep understanding of who you are and what you have to offer. Self-assurance is a reflection of masculine energy at its peak and a signal that you're willing to lead in the direction you choose.

Masculine energy is also the force that fuels passion and authenticity in your interactions. Passion for life, your goals, and your interests makes you magnetic. Women are attracted to passionate men, those who demonstrate an internal spark that lights their path and who also have a defined purpose. This has a lot to do with the previous chapter "live a unique life," as you may have noticed.

Authenticity, on the other hand, comes from alignment with your true self. Masculine energy drives you to be authentic and not hide your essence. Women perceive this as a valuable quality; you're real, different, authentic, honest, and this creates a deep, meaningful connection and will make women desire you more for who you are. Ultimately, knowing all this, it's now up to you to internalize your masculine energy and bring it to the surface if you haven't already.

To conclude the chapter, I want to invite you to reflection through a series of questions that will help you internalize the principles of masculine energy and, at the same time, help you acquire it if you don't have it yet. It's very important that you take a few minutes of your time now, in silence, to

reflect, grab a pen and paper, and take it very seriously. I've left space for you to write it down in the
same book if you wish.

1. How do you feel when interacting with someone who radiates confidence and security? Do you think this energy could impact your ability to attract other people, especially in the context of seduction?

2. Imagine someone who is in control of themselves and the situation, who walks with determination and confidence. What qualities of their energy do you find attractive, and how could you incorporate them into your own presence?

3. Have you ever experienced a conversation where you felt completely present, connected, and magnetic? What do you think contributed to that feeling, and how could you cultivate it more frequently?

4. Reflect on your past interactions. Are there moments when you feel that your energy or confidence diminished your chances of connection or attraction? What could you do differently in those situations?

5. Think of a leader you admire. What traits of their energy do you think make them a convincing leader? How could you incorporate some of those traits into your masculine energy?

6. How do you react to challenging or unfamiliar situations? Do you think your reaction could be influenced by your level of confidence and masculine energy?

7. Imagine what it would be like if you allowed yourself to express your desires and needs without fear of others' reactions. How do you think this could change the dynamics of your interactions and relationships?

8. What prevents you from being more authentic in your interactions? How do you think authenticity relates to masculine energy and its attractiveness in seduction?

9. Think of moments when you've felt insecure or nervous in social situations. What strategies could you use to calm those feelings and project a more secure and magnetic energy?

10. Visualize your most confident and at-
    tractive version. How do you walk?
    How do you talk? How do you hold
    yourself in challenging situations?
    What small steps could you take to
    move closer to that vision?

MASTER NONVERBAL COMMUNICATION: SOAR LIKE AN EAGLE

CHAPTER IX

Welcome to the next chapter, dear aspiring seducer, where we'll discuss the importance of nonverbal communication when it comes to seducing women. As you may have noticed on many occasions, not everything we want to convey is communicated verbally. In some circumstances, people tend to convey certain ideas or thoughts gesturally, whether through facial expressions, body gestures, or simply by stepping back from someone who makes them uncomfortable, indicating that their personal space is being invaded and they don't want any contact.

In the world of seduction, this is even more

important. Often, a woman won't directly tell you that she's attracted to you with her words, but rather indirectly through her gestures and body language. She might also tell you in the same way that she's not attracted to you. You must be very attentive and know how to interpret these signals in your favor, whether they are positive or negative. Once you've mastered this art, you'll know when to proceed and when to politely withdraw.

I warn you now... at first, interpreting these signals will be difficult, and it will require a great effort on your part to recognize them. But with practice, you'll come to do it automatically. It's like driving – it requires a lot of attention at first, but over time, you become accustomed to it and do it intuitively.

This chapter will be quite theoretical, which I don't particularly like, but I can't think of a better way to explain how nonverbal communication works. I believe it will be much easier to explain this way than with examples, and I want to ensure that you understand it clearly.

Next, I'm going to try to explain in detail the main gestures of a woman that indicate she's interested in you. So, get ready for pure theory!

<u>**Guide to Gestures Indicating a Woman Is Interested in You.**</u>

- **Sustained Eye Contact**: When a woman is interested, her gaze becomes one of her most powerful weapons. She will maintain prolonged eye contact with you and often seek your eyes repeatedly during the conversation. This gesture reveals a desire for connection and openness to intimacy.

- **Playful Smile**: Smiling is a key indicator of interest. Observe if her smile is genuine and radiant, especially when you are the center of her attention. An authentic smile shows that she feels comfortable and attracted to you.

- **Physical Proximity**: When a woman gets closer than necessary in a conversation, it can be a sign of interest. Pay attention to whether she leans toward you, lightly touches your arm, or creates a bubble of shared intimacy by reducing the distance between you.

- **Hair Play**: Women often play with their hair when they're interested. They may run their fingers through it, twist a lock, or play with their necklace or earrings.

This gesture is a manifestation of nervousness and flirtation.

- **Subtle Imitation**: If you notice her mirroring your gestures and postures, such as crossing her legs when you do, or taking a sip of her drink at the same time as you, it's a sign of harmony and connection. Subtle imitation indicates that she's tuning in to you at a deep level.

- **Touching Her Face or Lips**: An interesting gesture is when a woman gently touches her face or lips during the conversation. This may be an indication that she's contemplating the attraction she feels toward you and the possibility of desiring a kiss.

- **Leg Play**: Observe if she frequently crosses and uncrosses her legs while looking at you. This gesture can be a way to draw attention to her legs and express subtle interest.

Now that you know this, tiger, it's very important not to get ahead of yourself if you only identify one of these possible gestures. Keep calm. Typically, this works if you see about three to four signs and feel that the conversation is progressing and both of you are feeling comfortable. So, my advice, if you feel that the woman is making any of these gestures toward you but you're not sure if she likes you or not, wait to identify some more and continue with the conversation before trying anything else. You could also take a chance and see what happens, but you'll have a higher chance of failure, perhaps by moving too fast or being too forced. Or maybe you'll succeed... because who doesn't risk doesn't win. I'll leave this decision to you to act as you see fit.

To make it even clearer, I'm going to get technical with the negative gestures that indicate a woman is not interested in you, signaling that you need to leave the game and start anew. Because, yes, player! You don't always win...

Guide to Gestures Indicating a Woman Isn't Interested in You.

- **Limited or Avoidant Eye Contact**: One of the clearest signs of disinterest is a lack of eye contact or even avoiding looking at you. If she constantly looks around or down while talking, she's likely not interested in a romantic or flirtatious interaction.

- **Closed Body Posture**: When a woman crosses her arms over her chest or adopts a hunched posture, it may indicate discomfort or being closed off to interaction. This suggests a lack of willingness to connect.

- **Brief or Monosyllabic Responses**: If her answers are short and lacking detail, it's a sign she's not interested in engaging in meaningful conversation with you. It can be a way to express disinterest. Note that sometimes they may also test you this way to see how you react.

- **Lack of Initiative in Conversation**: If you're the one carrying the entire conversation and she doesn't contribute with topics or questions, she's likely not engaged in the interaction. She's showing lack of interest in you.

- **Physical Distance**: If she maintains significant distance between you, avoids physical contact, and backs away when you approach, it's a sign she's not comfortable with physical closeness. This indirectly indicates she's avoiding physical contact because in most cases she's not attracted to you, or not comfortable enough with you.

- **No Reaction to Touches or Compliments**: If you try to gently touch her arm or give her a compliment and she doesn't seem to react positively, it may indicate lack of interest or even discomfort in your presence.

- **Lack of Initiative to Continue Interaction**: When she shows no interest in continuing the interaction after an initial conversation, such as not asking for your number or not accepting an invitation for future meetings, it's a sign she's not interested in taking the relationship further. She might be trying to be polite with you in these cases, but she's not interested in you as a person; she's just being friendly.

- **Avoiding Personal Topics**: If she avoids discussing personal or emotional topics and sticks to superficial conversations, it may suggest she's not interested in deepening the connection. Alternatively, you may need to earn her trust for her to discuss more personal topics.

Congratulations! Now you know what the non-verbal signals, both positive and negative, indicate whether a woman is interested in you or not. But... what about you? As a man, you must know that you also subcommunicate through your gestures, confidence, or lack thereof, and as you have already learned in this book, what you want to communicate with your body language is confidence. So, I'm going to give you the keys below to know how you can communicate security with your body language.

Guide to Male Body Language: How to Convey Security or Insecurity

Projecting Security

- **Erect Posture**: Maintaining an upright posture with a straight back and shoulders back conveys confidence and self-esteem. Always show your best bearing. Remember that the first impression always comes through the eyes.

- **Firm Eye Contact**: Making direct and sustained eye contact shows that you are willing to face the situation with determination and sincerity. Remember, for my grandmother, seduction is done with looks. (She is not wrong at all).

- **Controlled Movements**: Controlled and deliberate gestures and movements indicate that you have control over yourself and your emotions. Gesturing gracefully while speaking could be an example. By gesturing, you indirectly capture their attention while communicating in a different way from others. This will make them pay more attention to you.

- **Relaxed Facial Expression**: A calm and serene facial expression suggests that you are in control of your emotions and comfortable with yourself. This means using your natural facial expression, without making strange grimaces or gestures that indicate you don't have the situation under control or show insecurity. (But remember, you can always make funny faces when joking around).

- **Firm and Clear Voice**: Speaking with a firm, clear, and confident voice is a powerful indicator of self-confidence. Make it clear that you are present! Without causing a scene.

<h1 style="text-align:center"><u>Projecting insecurity</u></h1>

- **Hunched or Stooped Posture**: A hunched posture, with shoulders slouched and head down, reflects insecurity and lack of confidence. This will make you blend into the background and most likely cause women not to notice you.

- **Avoiding Eye Contact**: Avoiding eye contact, or constantly looking down, can indicate discomfort or insecurity in the situation. Additionally, it indicates that you lack enough confidence in yourself to look someone in the eyes. (I'm not saying you should stare constantly and intensely into their eyes, as that would undoubtedly be quite uncomfortable. Instead, you should alternate, looking into their eyes, at their lips, or occasionally around you, but always look them in the eyes when they say something interesting or when you want to communicate something.)

- **Nervous Movements**: Repeatedly touching your hair, tapping your fingers, or fidgeting nervously can reveal anxiety or insecurity. (I'm not saying you shouldn't do these things. Personally, I sometimes like to tap my fingers, and there's nothing wrong with it at all. However, doing it constantly and accompanied by other possible gestures of the same kind can demonstrate insecurity.)

- **Tense Facial Expression**: A tense facial expression, with furrowed brow or signs of anxiety, suggests lack of confidence in the situation. As we've already discussed, the key is to be natural; maintain the same facial expression you would with your best friend. With practice, you'll learn to use a more seductive facial expression.

- **Trembling or Hesitant Voice**: Speaking with a trembling or hesitant voice indicates insecurity and lack of self-assurance. The same goes for speaking with a very soft tone of voice. By doing this, you subcommunicate that you don't want anyone to hear what you're saying or doing.

To finish off this chapter, let's move on to another personal anecdote of mine. You know I love sharing them, and luckily, I have plenty to tell. A few days ago, I went out in my hometown. (You might be thinking, "Wasn't he in Switzerland?" Well, I was, but right now I'm rewriting this chapter, and yes, I returned to Valencia a few days ago, with the intention of staying for at least a while. I'll see if I go back to Switzerland, or if I become a millionaire by writing this book. Fingers crossed.)

But I digress again. I was with some friends as usual, having a drink to change things up. (I love beer, rum and coke, and a good Old Fashioned.) You don't need to drink to flirt, but I enjoy a drink when I go out, so I got into the groove. (From my point of view, there's nothing wrong with having a drink to flirt, as long as you don't overdo it. However, I emphasize that it's not necessary. Personally, I enjoy drinking moderately, so I'm being myself.)

After a while, we got tired of the bar where we were with my friends, so we decided to go to a nightclub in the city center. We went in, everything was normal, and we formed the typical circle of friends. I started to look around, as usual, seeking knowing glances and analyzing what was around me while chatting and dancing with my friends.

Observing the surroundings, I noticed a blonde girl with fair skin and blue eyes, quite attractive and tall. She was dancing with another man, but I felt like she was looking at me, so I decided to wink at her, while giving her a mischievous smile. (This would confirm whether she was looking at me or not.) Sure enough, she saw me, laughed, and moved away a bit from the other man, as if waiting for me to come and talk or dance with her.

The truth is, I was having a good time with my friends, the night had just begun, and I didn't feel like talking to her at that moment, so I decided to let the opportunity pass for the time being. But about an hour later, after this happened, my friends told me they were leaving. Since I didn't feel like going home yet, I decided to stay alone in the club, with the idea that I might not end up going home alone if I played my cards right.

I said goodbye to my friends, raised my gaze again, looked around, and saw the girl I had been exchanging glances with. She was still dancing with the other man, but I was sure he hadn't kissed her yet. I noticed she moved away a bit and went to the bar to get something. It was my moment to act!

I gather my courage and head to the bar. I position myself next to her, greet her with a smile, and then mention that I noticed she had been looking at me. She confirms it and laughs shyly. I suggest changing dance partners, to which she laughs again and tells me she's not going to go with a Playboy like me to play with her. I laugh even more and tell her what makes her think I'm a Playboy. She responds, "The way you look at me and the words you said when you talked to me." Additionally, she adds that the other guy was treating her very well and she felt bad about ditching him for me.

Throughout this exchange, she continued to look at me with desire; I could feel it. Moreover, she kept smiling at me and maintained quite a close distance from me. I felt that she was interested. Otherwise, she wouldn't have bothered to spend so much time with me.

I pondered for a moment and then said, "Look, the difference between that man and me is that at least I'm straightforward with you and tell you what I think and want. Plus, I can guarantee you that by the end of the night, that other guy will want the same thing I want now."

She was surprised but also seemed to like my response. She said, "I'll talk to the other man too, so I can decide what I want. Wait for me here." I agreed to the deal and went to get a beer.

The girl returns to me; it was clear she liked me. She couldn't stop smiling at me, looking into my eyes, and always staying close to me. Suddenly, she confesses that she was more attracted to me than the other guy simply because of how I approached her. However, she also admits that she felt bad for the other guy.

We continue with this nonsensical conversation for a while until I get tired and kiss her because I knew she liked it. She reciprocates and kisses me back. Suddenly, she stops talking about the other man, and we start talking about us. (Here I had to take the leap to show my intentions and end the game.)

Throughout this, the other guy kept watching us, but he hadn't been lucky enough to read Giovanni Amato's advice, like you're doing now. What could the poor guy do? I felt sorry for him. But I would have felt even worse going home alone. So, I continued with my game.

I spent another hour dancing and kissing her, and I suggested going somewhere together. She tells me I could go to her caravan with her, but we had to wait for her friend. What a nightmare! It was hard to convince her friend to leave; she was a bit drunk and didn't want to leave alone, out of envy for her friend, I suppose. That's another story, but in the end, I did it.

Finally, I ended up in the caravan with both of them. Unfortunately, there was no threesome, if that's what you're thinking, but there was a duo. Moreover, I spent that weekend with them, traveling along the Valencian coast and sleeping on the beach. It was a crazy plan that I wouldn't have had if I hadn't approached that girl in the nightclub.

I must confess that I quite liked the girl, and I would have liked to join their trip. In fact, they invited me to travel with them. However, I'm currently strapped for cash and couldn't afford it. In case you're curious, they told me they would pass through Valencia again to see me, but personally, even if it does happen, I don't like getting my hopes up for these things (for the sake of my mental health, mostly). If it happens, great, and if not, that's fine too. (Update: It didn't happen; at that moment, I was meeting another girl and didn't have time to meet with her). What a shame.

But the experience was fantastic, and now I'm sharing it with you, hoping it serves as a learning experience for you.

I believe that with all this theory, you will understand how women communicate attraction without saying a word and how men convey confidence through body language. It's crucial that you understand all of this before moving on to the next chapter, where you'll learn how to initiate a successful conversation with a woman.

It's very important that the next time you go out, you pay close attention to these small details. Therefore, I want to propose a series of simple exercises for you to do next time you go out. They will help you identify these gestures more easily and internalize them so that you can recognize them automatically.

<u>Exercise:</u>

1. **Go to a social environment** where you know there is interaction between men and women, such as a bar, nightclub, or café. Observe while having a drink how men and women interact. Pay special attention to the non-verbal communication mentioned earlier. Try to identify positive and negative verbal communication. Also, try to identify if the man conveys confidence or insecurity with his body language, and reflect on it. If necessary, jot down notes in a notebook. Analyze it as if you were a seduction teacher wanting to teach your student.

2. **Movie Analysis**: I'm going to suggest a series of titles where non-verbal communication focused on seduction is clear, so you can also reflect as in the previous exercise, but this time from the comfort of your home. The movies are as follows:

- **"Hitch"**: is a film that introduces a "dating doctor" who uses non-verbal communication strategies to help others conquer their romantic interests. It provides funny and practical examples of how to use body language in seduction situations.

- **"Crazy, Stupid, Love"**: This movie focuses on how a character who is an expert in seduction shares his knowledge and techniques with others. It offers clear examples and lessons on body language, style, and self-confidence.

- **"Two and a Half Men"**: While not as focused on seduction, it also includes clear scenes of non-verbal communication, both positive and negative, between its two main characters. Plus, it will give you some laughs.

3. **Personal Reflection**: Try to recall interactions you've had with women in the past and remember how their non-verbal communication was. Was it positive or negative? On your part, did you display confidence or insecurity with your body? Identify the principles listed above in each situation and write them down if you think it's necessary. The goal of this exercise is for you to reflect on your past interactions so you can improve your non-verbal communication skills and interpret female non-verbal communication.

THE ART OF STARTING A CONVERSATION

Now that you have understood and internalized the art of non-verbal communication, let's take the next step, Dr. Love. In this chapter, you will learn how you can initiate a conversation with any woman you set your sights on and succeed, or at least give it a try and not die trying.

I imagine you still feel afraid and insecure about approaching that woman you like. Don't worry, we'll solve it together. If it's any consolation, let me remind you that I too was unable to approach and talk to a woman. I was a coward, didn't want to admit it, and didn't believe in myself. That was the main problem. Let's get straight to the point.

One of the most common mistakes men make when they want to interact with a woman is that they idolize them. They put them on a pedestal and think they're goddesses from Olympus, descended from the heavens. Unattainable to mortal eyes, so the man assumes his role as a mere mortal and avoids interaction at all costs because of the idea he has put in his head. As you can imagine, this is nothing more than nonsense from an insecure man who still doesn't know what he wants, isn't aware of his worth, and has no idea what women are like.

My intention is for you to lose that irrational fear you have in your head of starting a conversation with a woman because, even if you don't believe me yet, it's much easier than it seems. Let me tell you a little secret: women are dying to receive attention from a man. They love it, like a junkie loves cocaine. It motivates them, makes them feel better, and generally desired. I also tell you that personally, as a seducer, I love receiving attention from a woman. It boosts my ego and makes me feel desired. Who wouldn't want that? But I also believe that many men are not aware of this.

Knowing that women love to receive attention, we start from a clear advantage: they desire attention, and you are eager to talk to that girl you like. Perfect, but obviously it's not that easy because they also don't want the attention of just any man. Generally speaking, they want the attention of a high-value man, a wolf, not a lamb. Hence the importance of the previous chapters, which will have helped you gain more confidence in yourself or at least opened your eyes to what you need to do to gain it.

Continuing with this explanation, doesn't everything start to make more sense? The woman seeks the attention of a man with masculine energy, who is confident and has good vibes. Great! You are a man who is reading this book to make a change in his life, discovering knowledge that you didn't have until today, working on being a better version of yourself, more confident, and therefore, if you achieve this, you will be more desired in the eyes of a woman. So what's stopping you from talking to that woman? She is eager for you to talk to her, she wants your attention, she wants to feel desired, she wants you to boost her ego. So start playing!

Fantastic, you've realized it, and now you've had the guts to go talk to her. She smiled at you, but you're blank because you don't know what to say, you lack practice. It's okay. Let it flow, ask her about her likes, her hobbies, show interest in getting to know her. At first, it's normal to force the conversation a bit; the important thing is that she responds to you and asks you back. Breaking the ice is crucial here. Don't forget to pay attention to the non-verbal communication I mentioned earlier.

Congratulations! You've reached the first step;

you're sitting at the bar talking to that beautiful woman, but you feel forced and still don't know what to expect from the conversation. That's because you don't have a defined action plan.

Now let me tell you another secret: to seduce a woman in one night or during the day, you don't need hours of conversation to get her attention. Just making the conversation flow, making her laugh, is enough to take the next step; show her your intentions. Ask for her number if you meet on the street, or propose sitting down for a coffee, under the pretext of getting to know each other better. You could use the typical example of something about her that caught your attention and that you would like to get to know her for that reason, either at that moment or another. Since this is not a book of canned phrases and copy and paste, I prefer you to use your wit when the occasion arises. With practice, you'll come up with better lines, of course, after messing up a few times. Don't expect success in your first attempts.

If you're at a bar or a nightclub, suggest going dancing or ask her for a kiss directly. The worst that can happen is that she says no, and you will gracefully step back with a smile. You're in luck because you're not a medieval knight who has to maintain his honor intact, and you can afford to be rejected.

Knowing this, I'm going to tell you another

personal story to motivate you because I like telling stories, listening to them, and because it's my book, and I feel like telling you, and because if you want to be a good seducer, you'll also have to tell good stories from time to time.

A few months ago, I was at a bar in Lausanne, Switzerland, one night. I had finished my shift as a bartender, so I felt like having a drink to relax from work. I arrived at the bar, had a couple of beers with a friend. We were talking about life and how to progress in it and how to leave that job that we didn't like but was currently paying my rent.

As the conversation flowed with my friend, I looked up and saw a woman looking at me. She was an Asian woman, quite attractive, fair-skinned, with black hair, dark eyes, and a bit tall for a woman, she definitely caught my attention and that of a few others.

I gave her a slight smile, and she returned it, so I decided to get up and go talk to her. I approached her, said a simple "Hello" in English, and then said, "I noticed we were looking at each other, and I wanted to know if it was just me or if you were really looking at me." She said, "It's true, I was looking at you." I laughed with a mischievous smile and replied, "What, do you like looking at me like that?" And she responded, "Well, you don't look bad," and she laughed too.

Seems pretty easy, right? Then I invited her to

dance, and we danced a bit, to music that wasn't exactly to my taste (don't think I'm a good dancer either, the other day they laughed at how I danced), but the important thing was to move a little, get closer to her, and see that she wasn't uncomfortable with my presence. Indeed, she let me get closer, looked me in the eyes, and smiled all the time, so I decided, without much thought, to kiss her, which she eagerly returned as we continued dancing.

I thought everything was done, but suddenly, something strange happened that I must confess had never happened to me in my entire life. I must also confess that I didn't really care because all I wanted at that moment was to sleep with her.

Returning to the story, this girl said to me, "Giovanni, I was with another guy I like before, and I want to see who kisses better to decide whether to go with him or with you." I was quite surprised, to which I responded, "Well, do what you have to do, I'm not going to wait for you, but let me know how it goes."

Indeed, she kissed this other guy, came back, and I asked, "So, who kisses better then?" She said it was the other guy. I laughed, told her to go with him then, and she said, "No, I like you more, I see you as more confident, and I want to go with you tonight." So, we had one more beer at that place and then went to my room since I currently share a house. (I didn't kiss her again until she brushed her teeth at my place.) We had a good night, and we continued seeing each other for a while without any commitment until she went back to her home country, Mongolia.

As you may have noticed if you paid attention to this little personal story, sometimes you don't need to say great things or have a magnificent entrance to get the attention of that woman you like. Sometimes, all it takes is to act and show confidence in yourself.

I am aware that many gurus teach openers on how to start a conversation, but in my personal opinion, those openers often don't work because you won't be able to say and convey them naturally since they are not your inventions but just a copy and paste of what someone said someday, and it will show.

That's why, for me, it's better to go straight and simply say whatever comes to your mind. I'm sure you'll make many mistakes and find yourself in embarrassing situations on your own, but you need to go through that, my friend, as being a seducer will require a lot of practice and many embarrassing situations.

Next, I'll leave you with a guide for you to refer to as many times as you need, in which I detail the steps to start a conversation with that girl you like.

Step-by-step guide to initiate a successful conversation

- **Make eye contact**: As discussed in the previous chapter, paying attention to non-verbal cues is crucial. If a girl is looking at you, she's likely interested in getting to know you. It's usually your job to approach and start a conversation with her. While it's not always necessary to have eye contact to initiate a conversation, it often helps. I've initiated conversations without prior eye contact and ended up spending the night with her, but having eye contact beforehand can certainly make things easier.

- **Break the ice**: Remember that women are waiting for the attention of a man and to feel desired to boost their ego, and because we all seek companionship. Keep this in mind whenever you want to approach a woman to boost your own confidence and not let your fears take over. You don't need to say the most clever phrase to start a conversation with a woman who caught your attention. In most cases, simply starting the conversation in a way that makes you feel confident is enough. So don't think twice and go talk to her; remember that

it's better to try than to regret not trying.

- **Be yourself, stay natural**: Don't pretend
to be someone you're not to flirt. Stay
true to yourself, try to be funny, show
security, and confidence in yourself.

- **Show interest in her**: Avoid talking all
the time about yourself, as it can bore
them. Instead, show interest in her, ask
about her life, her hobbies, in short, take
the time to get to know her. Try to spark
her interest and make her ask about you
too. If you notice that the conversation
flows, there are smiles, she looks at you,
and there's a good vibe, it's time to take
the next step, buddy.

- **Show your intentions**: This is where
many men fail, including myself at first.
Sometimes we focus so much on the
conversation and making a good impression that we forget about our intentions. That's why it's essential to always
be clear about your intentions and show
them as soon as you feel a connection. If
you're attracted to her and want to have
a good time, give her a kiss or take it further, you have to tell her and show her
what you feel. Don't say it right away,
but pay attention to the conversation,

and when you feel like you can't hold back what you feel anymore, don't hesitate and simply say it.

Now that you know the step-by-step process for initiating a successful conversation, let's focus on how to keep the conversation going so that the girl doesn't get bored, and you can achieve your goal.

<u>**Simple strategies to maintain the conversation**</u>

- **Ask Open-Ended Questions**: Instead of asking closed-ended questions that only require yes or no answers, ask open-ended questions that encourage more detailed responses and deeper conversation. For example, instead of asking "Do you like to travel?", you can ask "What has been your favorite travel destination and why?".

- **Listen Actively**: Pay attention to what the other person is saying. Don't interrupt or jump ahead with your own responses while listening. Ask follow-up questions based on what you heard to show that you're interested.

- **Share Personal Stories**: Sharing personal anecdotes related to the conversation topic can make the conversation more intimate and meaningful. Personal stories allow the other person to get to know you better. Tell stories about that trip you enjoyed so much, or something funny that happened with your friends recently.

- **Vary the Topics**: Avoid getting stuck on one topic for too long. Change the subject naturally when you feel the conversation is running out of steam. This keeps the conversation fresh and exciting. You can always return to previous topics, as there are always things left to say.

- **Use Humor**: Humor is an excellent way to lighten the mood and make the conversation more engaging. Don't force jokes, but if an opportunity for a funny comment arises, don't hesitate to seize it. Women love funny men, don't forget.

- **Speak with Passion**: If you talk about something you're truly passionate about, your enthusiasm will be contagious. Share your interests and passions, and the other person will likely be drawn to your enthusiasm. Talk about your latest trip, the project you're working on, a funny situation you experienced, or anything that excites you.

- **Show Interest**: Ask about the other person's interests, hobbies, and goals, and show genuine interest in getting to know them better. People tend to enjoy conversations when they feel that the other person cares about them.

- **Use Appropriate Body Language**: Body language plays an important role in communication. Maintain eye contact, smile, and use gestures that reinforce what you're saying.

- **Listen to the Other Person's Signals**: Pay attention to the other person's non-verbal cues. If they seem bored or uncomfortable, consider changing the topic or adjusting your approach to the conversation. Or if they don't like the place where you are, try going somewhere else.

- **Be Authentic**: Most importantly, be yourself. Authenticity is attractive, and people enjoy genuine conversations. Don't try to be someone you're not to impress someone. They'll eventually figure it out, and you'll end up worse off.

Remember that this is mere theory and it will be worthless if you don't put it into practice in the following days after reading this chapter. Therefore, I'm going to propose a series of exercises for you to put into practice what you've learned and so you can soon become the next Leonardo DiCaprio.

<u>Exercise:</u>

1. **Attend a language exchange event**. It's a simple idea, you can go wherever you want to practice, but I think it's a good option. Generally, women who attend these types of events are predisposed to conversation and you can also practice what you've learned, as well as learn a new language. Look online for a bar in your city that hosts these kinds of events; they are usually called "language exchange."

2. **Meet up with a trusted friend**. If you don't feel comfortable doing it alone, suggest to a friend who also wants to learn how to converse and flirt, to go to a bar or shopping center and start conversations with strangers. This way, you won't feel alone and you'll have moral support in case the conversation doesn't go as expected. If you don't have any interested friends, gather up the courage to do it on your own.

3. **Join a group related to your favorite hobby**. This way, you'll be engaging in an activity that you're passionate about, and you'll know that the other person also shares your interests, making it easier for you to start a conversation

with a common topic of interest. If you
don't have a hobby, try to think about
what you enjoy and look for something
related to that.

THAWING OUT: CONQUERING MENTAL BLOCKS

CHAPTER XI

The dreaded mental block, undoubtedly one of the greatest enemies of the seducer, and even more so of the aspiring one. From my humble opinion, it's something that will always be within us. Impossible to shake off, but definitely possible to overcome.

I confess that even today, I occasionally feel this damn block when I want to initiate an interaction from scratch. Luckily for me, I know the principles to unblock myself and continue with the inter-action, so in this chapter, I'll share those principles with you.

But first, what causes this recurring mental

block in all men and seducers? Primarily, it's due to a human defense mechanism to avoid embarrassing or uncomfortable situations since, as you know, humans tend to favor comfort and routine. However, this defense mechanism doesn't help us at all when it comes to seducing a woman. We need to learn to control it for successful relationships; we need to let it go. Otherwise, if you can't overcome it, you'll always be an insecure guy, unable to approach and talk to a girl, and you'll spend your life frustrated, wondering why you're always alone.

First of all, let's study the main fears that cross our minds and sabotage that initial interaction, leaving us paralyzed and unable to act.

There are four main blocks that affect the male mind, which I'll enumerate now. I'll be brief here because in my previous book, "Seductive Mindset: Attract, Seduce, Conquer," I delve into greater detail and explain it very clearly. If you haven't read it yet and feel you need to delve deeper into this topic, or simply want to support me and help me earn some royalties to fully dedicate myself to this, I suggest you purchase it. Let's get down to business.

<u>**The Four Great Enemies of the Seducer.**</u>

1. **Fear of What Others Will Say Block**: Sometimes, we're terrified of what others might think of us. You must understand that this is nothing more than a defense mechanism of an insecure lamb. If we analyze it coldly, it's just a load of crap that prevents us from doing what we really want, out of a fear that isn't real. I can assure you that most of the time, even if you've been rejected, others will admire you for having the courage to go for it, as it's well-known that many men don't even dare to take the first step. So, in short... forget about the rest and focus on yourself, not just for seduction but for achieving any goal you set for yourself. Uncomfortable situations often make us stronger. Seize the opportunity!

2. **Fear of Rejection**: Many men are afraid of the simple possibility of being rejected by a woman. They think they'll be less, they'll be judged, or any other mental nonsense that comes to mind. I'm sorry, dear reader, rejection is something that can never be controlled. It's just another factor in the equation of this seduction game and will always be

a possible outcome or variable. So, you have to accept it and play your cards accordingly. There's no trick to overcoming this fear; you simply have to understand that it's part of the game, not let it affect you when this variable arises, and most importantly, not let it block you. Accepting that rejection will always be present is key to making sure it doesn't affect you. If you know in advance that there's a chance you'll be rejected and still take the risk, with practice, you'll eventually stop caring. Don't be proud. Accept rejection. Your life won't end just because you're rejected!

3. **The Self-Saboteur**: By this, I mean the predisposition to failure with which one begins an interaction or doesn't even start it. (Mindset). Many men tend to think that it won't go well for them before they've even tried. And indeed, it doesn't go well because they were predisposed with that mindset before anything even happened. This tends to happen due to negative experiences in the past. But here's the thing: you want to be a wolf, so you have to change that mindset and forget about it. You already know that the worst thing that can happen is rejection, which you al-

ready knew. Don't sabotage yourself with negative thoughts; instead, approach the game with an open mind. Forget about your own personal prejudices and simply take action, talk to her, and see what happens. You already have the "no"!

4. **Fear of Not Being Good Enough Block**: This fear comes hand in hand with lack of self-confidence. I won't go into much detail here, as I've dedicated several chapters previously to this topic and how to overcome it. So, I imagine you already have an idea.

Knowing that all of this is the most normal thing on planet Earth, and that even the most experienced seducer in the world occasionally gets overwhelmed by these fears, let's focus on how you can overcome them.

I want you to draw your own conclusions, so I'll leave the keys and principles to overcome them in the following story. Since the block will always appear sooner or later, it's important to admit it, and once recognized, be aware and not let it take over. Let me explain it better in this little story.

Last weekend, I was in a bar in Valencia with some friends. You might say, "Damn, this guy is bar-hopping!" The truth is, yeah, maybe I have a problem with drinking... (Just kidding.) The fact is, I've always believed that the best atmosphere for flirting is a bar, as people are generally more sociable and receptive to starting a conversation with a stranger. (Plus, I want to dedicate myself to this, so I always look for scenarios to put my knowledge into practice; otherwise, I wouldn't have anything to tell you.)

So, I was with some friends who aren't very good at flirting, let's not lie, and after a couple of drinks... my body was craving some interaction with a woman. For simple fun, to get a bit of adrenaline pumping, and because let's be honest, I don't like sleeping alone, no point in deceiving anyone.

The thing is, at the table next to us, there was a group of four pretty attractive women. But I have to confess that I was sabotaging myself a bit because I kept telling myself: "Your friends aren't good at flirting, half of them have girlfriends and won't be interested in playing along. There are four of them and just one of you. It probably won't go well, maybe they'll be annoyed, and most likely, my friends won't help me in the interaction. So maybe it's better not to even try because chances are I won't get anything out of it."

I had this idea in my head for a while, until I thought to myself again: "Who cares about all that! If you feel like it, go and talk to them. In the end, you know the worst that can happen is they don't want to talk to you, so I'll just go back to my friends, politely withdraw, and no harm done." Besides, personally, I hate the feeling of 'what if...' I prefer to be rejected than to be left wondering.

In the end, I went with my last thought, so I stood up, approached their table, and said:
    - Hey, what's the plan for tonight?
    - We don't know yet, what do you suggest?
    - For now, we can have a drink and get to know each other. How does that sound?
    - Sure, sounds great. (They said with laughter).

I was wearing a Valencia shirt as I had just come from the football stadium. So they asked me how they could go there. I told them they could buy tickets online and next time they should come with us to the stadium. I also asked if I could sit with them, to which they gladly accepted.

At first, I didn't know exactly what to say, I was a bit nervous, don't ask me why, but sometimes it happens to me, so I decided to resort to the typical questions asked when starting a conversation. "Where are you from? How long have you been here? What do you do with your life?" And all that. I also took advantage of the football topic to propose some future plans, which although may not materialize, everyone likes to talk about a different plan. In this case, it was going to the stadium together. (Sometimes it's a good idea to propose future plans to see if they're interested in getting to know you or not). (Valencia plays in 2 weeks, and since I have their Instagram, I can always propose the plan if I feel like it). (Update, the plan never happened, but as I've said many times, the important thing here is to enjoy the moment).

It turned out they were Italian and were doing their aesthetics internship in my hometown. The conversation was going quite well, and they began to show interest in me, asking personal questions to which I responded gracefully, and they seemed to enjoy the conversation. It seemed like it was going to be a night where I wouldn't be sleeping alone.

Meanwhile, my friends were at another table, so I invited them to join the conversation, and we all started sharing that moment. Trying to give the best version of ourselves without forgetting to enjoy the moment, we spent about an hour chatting, having a good time.

At the end of the night, the girls had to leave as they had internships the next day, so I asked the one I liked for her Instagram. In a fun way, I told her it would be a way to stay in touch when they came to see the football match, and that I would show them how to have a good pre-game with the fans. She gladly accepted and gave me her Instagram. The night ended, and I went home alone. No matter how good you are, you don't always win. But I also say that if you always won, this game wouldn't be fun.

To finish the story, I must confess that I messaged her on Instagram yesterday, saying that I would like to meet up with her alone for a drink and get to know each other better. She responded that she had a boyfriend, but we could all meet up again for a drink another day. I said yes, we had a good time, why not repeat it another day?

In the end, what's important is that you can't control everything. In seduction, you have to adapt to what happens. Even though I would have loved to spend the night with her or to meet her again alone to flirt with her, she has a boyfriend, or so she says. I don't know if it's true or if it's an excuse because she's not interested, but it's something I can't control, and I must accept it as it is. After all, I had a good night, and I have the opportunity to meet her and her friends again... and who knows? Maybe I can flirt with someone else. And if not, life goes on... and luckily, there are many women to meet.

In conclusion, I hope you've come to the realization that the block is nothing more than a mental nonsense that will prevent you from experiencing at least a fun situation because of an unfounded fear. Knowing that in the best-case scenario, you might end up not sleeping alone that night, or in the worst case, you might be ignored. But... are you going to miss the opportunity to find out what could happen because of a simple fear that isn't real? Perhaps the next woman of your life is at the next table, and because of your fear or block, you'll miss the chance to meet her, and you won't have it ever again.

Don't let the block paralyze you. If this happens, resort to typical questions to get through it. With practice, you'll develop your own methods to get out of this situation quickly. Practice makes perfect!

A quick tip before finishing the chapter that helped me a lot to overcome the block was the following: when I felt intimidated inside and blocked at first, I always told myself, "If you don't go, someone else will, and you'll miss the opportunity, giving another man a chance." Or, she'll just leave, and you'll never see her again. Believe me, there's nothing more frustrating than watching the girl you like at the party leave with another guy, while you stand there looking like a fool.

<u>**Practical Guide to Overcoming Blockages in Your Next Interaction**</u>

1. **Social Blockage**: When you're afraid of what others might think, remember that by gathering courage and starting the interaction, even in the worst-case scenario of rejection, people around you will see you as a courageous man because you had the guts to try while they didn't. Men will admire you, and women will be attracted to you!

2. **Rejection**: Something you can't control. Accept that you'll never have a 100% success rate. (Not even Brad Pitt has it, well maybe he does... but you weren't born with that legendary skin). Accept rejection as a part of the equation. Who doesn't risk, doesn't win, so don't leave with doubts. It's worse to wonder what could have happened if... than facing rejection. Realize this, and you'll thank me in the future. You want to be a seducer, so accept this as part of the game. I didn't invent the rules; it's an unwritten universal law, so you're not going to change it now. Embrace the game.

3. **Fear of Failure**: Every time your mind tells you that you're going to fail, remember that it's a possibility, but if you don't try, someone else will, and they'll steal the girl you like. Do you want to see how she gets stolen? Or would you prefer to try and at least leave with the peace of mind that you didn't stand there like a fool, fantasizing about her naked body and the self-pleasure you'll do at home? Self-pleasure will always be waiting for you at home... so try not to be loyal to your hand. Cheat on it with a real woman. I'm sure it'll forgive you and won't take it personally.

4. **Self-Motivation Factor**: You're reading this book because I imagine you're tired of spending nights alone, not having a partner, and meeting few women. The next time you're blocked, think of the following: "I'm not Brad Pitt, so women won't come to me. If I don't want to sleep alone again tonight, I'll have to gather some courage and go talk to her, otherwise, I'll end up masturbating again."

Try to memorize this so that every time you feel blocked, you can overcome it and take action. But always keep in mind that blockage is just a mental trick, mostly unfounded by a fear that is often imaginary. So... the next time it happens to you, will you let yourself be ruled by your blockage? Or on the contrary, will you realize how absurd it is and take action? You might even meet your Angelina Jolie. Would you miss the opportunity because of a simple blockage? In the worst-case scenario, you'll know who will comfort you when you get home alone...

PLAN B: YOUR SECRET WEAPON

CHAPTER XII

Having a plan B ready will be one of the best things you can do if you want to succeed on a date. By this, I mean always having in mind a place to take the girl after a date, whether you've hooked up at the club or any other scenario that comes to mind. But it's super crucial if you want to seal the deal and take her to bed.

I want to make a brief chapter about this, as the other day, I was on vacation in my hometown, Valencia. In case you're curious, I currently live in Switzerland, although I'm considering moving back to Spain. But anyway, I digress, and that's another story. I'm telling you this to provide some context and earn your trust, so you see that I'm just a normal person trying to make a living by writing.

Let me tell you the story. As I mentioned, I was in Valencia, my hometown, but I hadn't rented any hotel or anything. So, I found myself sleeping at my parents' house. I have many sisters, and the house is quite full, plus my parents are very conservative and don't like it much if I bring any woman home.

I decided to go out that night with a friend. We went out for dinner, a burger if I remember correctly, and then we decided to go grab a drink to warm up for the club. Everything was going great so far. We went to the club, talked for a while, had a few more drinks, took a stroll to see the people and the women around. We were having a good time, dancing, laughing, you know, what you do in a club.

This club I'm talking about is quite big, it's called MYA, and it has plenty of rooms and terraces. As we were walking around, I saw a girl I liked, who was sitting on a terrace with her friend. She caught my eye, so I decided to make a move. I approached her, greeted her, looked her in the eyes, smiled (with a seductive and mischievous smile), introduced myself, and asked if she minded me joining them. They gave me permission, so I sat down, and we started talking. She was from the United States, I don't remember which city, and typically, she spoke English, but also a little bit of Spanish, so we spoke both languages.

There was quite a bit of chemistry, and the attraction was palpable. In the midst of all this, I was a bit drunk and accidentally knocked over my glass, spilling it all over the table. I looked clumsy, but we laughed it off, and it was like nothing had happened. (Making a fool of yourself is natural, so sometimes it can even boost confidence. Don't let yourself be carried away by an embarrassing situation, and resolve it naturally by downplaying its importance.)

The only issue was that her friend wasn't very talkative and attractive, so my friend wasn't really engaged in the conversation with her. It wasn't flowing, so to speak. The friend wanted to move to another area of the club, so I asked for her Instagram, she gave it to me, and we each went our separate ways.

So far, so good. Normal. There's interest. I'm with my friend, I know the girl likes me, and I knew I would run into her again later in the same club. So, I acted indifferent, with the assurance that I would see her again.

Sure enough, I bumped into her about an hour later. I approached her, we talked again, danced, I asked for a little kiss, she gave it to me, but once again, her friend got bored and decided she wanted to leave. Since they came together, they'd leave together. I insisted a bit, joked that they were tourists and should stay to enjoy the night, but it didn't work, and they left. Nothing new or surprising, she said, "You have my Instagram, we'll stay in touch."

Great, I text her later, saying the usual, "It was great meeting you, I had a good time, but I was hoping to spend the night with you," hit send, and that was it. She responded that she felt the same and would love to have a good night with me, but she needed to be picked up.

Since that night, I preferred to hook up than stay in the club, I hailed a taxi and went to get her. On the way, I realized I didn't have a damn place to take her, so I improvised and told myself, "I have to play the rooftop card." It was too late to rent a hotel, I couldn't go to my parents' house, and hers was also out of the question because she was with a host family.

Life's little curveballs. I go to her place, she comes down, we start walking towards mine, and feeling guilty, I decide to be honest and tell her the plan. I tell her I'm staying with my parents, that I live in Switzerland, that I don't have a place here, and that the idea was to go to the rooftop.

Obviously, she's not thrilled about the idea of having sex outdoors. I tell her it's not the first time I've done it (I screw up even more). She says she's not going there, that she thought I had a place, and that's why she was going to come with me, so she decides to stay at her host family's house instead.

She gives me a kiss, we agree to meet another day, and I go back alone to my parents' house, thinking that at least I got a chapter out of this experience for my book. So, that's something.

Summary and reflection. I never saw the girl again because I went back to Switzerland, which is a shame because she was a real beauty in my eyes. The reflection is that no matter how experienced or good you are at seducing, some women won't go anywhere with you if you don't have a place to take them.

That's why it's crucial if you plan to have something more on a random night or any date, you need to have at least some place to take her, other than a rooftop. Even though I've done it before, not all women are willing to go to a place like that, especially if they're beautiful, value themselves, and come from the United States.

In conclusion, dear reader, never forget the importance of having a good place to take them, or you'll end up regretting it like I did that night. I admit that on this occasion, I had to be comforted by my friend "Mast." A great pity, considering the opportunity I missed with that beauty, just because I didn't have a place to take her.

PART III:

Mastering Seduction:
Elevate Your Seduction Game
to the Next Level.

LOVE: THE ULTIMATE DESIRE

It might seem like an obvious statement, but it holds great truth. Everyone, and I repeat, everyone needs companionship and love in their lives. No one wants to spend their life alone. It's true that sometimes it's great to know how to be alone, to make the most of your time and engage in solo activities. But at the end of the day, you always want to have someone to share your time with and tell them about your day. Because the truth is, we are social beings and we need human interaction to be happy.

When we relate this to seduction, the key here is to understand that all women who are not in a relationship, generally speaking, will be seeking companionship, whether it's a boyfriend, a friend with benefits, or someone to spend the night with.

Keeping this in mind will give you an advantage. I know many people who don't even consider this, or who simply aren't aware of this great truth.

Furthermore, in this era of social media and virtual communication, many people are feeling more alone than ever. We all see perfect lives on social media, which in reality are not so perfect, but it leads us to overthink and believe that our lives aren't as perfect, that we don't have as many friends as others, or as many women as that person. This often leads to comparison, in a spiral that is very harmful to our mental health, causing feelings of loneliness to surface in our minds. This applies to both women and men.

The irony is that we are more connected than ever, yet never before in the history of humanity have people felt such a need to create real connections, to avoid falling into the void of vanity and loneliness.

So, a piece of advice I give you is to forget about social media a bit. Use it as a tool to maintain contact, but focus more on the real world. Meet women in the offline world, this will help you create more real, true, and lasting connections.

Returning to the topic of seeking companionship related to seduction. The important thing is to understand that everyone seeks to interact with others, all single women are looking for that guy who will take them out of their monotony. If you can understand this, it will be much easier for you to start an interaction with that girl who has caught your attention. If you play your cards right, you can touch her emotional chord and fill that void of companionship with your presence. If you achieve this, I guarantee she will be yours. You will have successfully seduced her and most likely secure another date.

This is something I now share with you in a very simple way, but it has taken me years to understand, and therefore, this is a key element to seducing in the most natural way possible.

But beware, here you have to be careful not to play with the other person's feelings by taking advantage of this principle. First, out of respect, and secondly, because I'm telling you from experience, if you take too much advantage of this, karma will come back to you, and I say this because it has happened to me. Be careful, because this truth is a double-edged sword that should not be used with malice but with naturalness. It's important to remember that seducing is one thing and deceiving is another. As a seducer, your goal should be for both her and you to have a pleasant time, based on respect, honesty, and naturalness. (You can also add a touch of mischief). So use this to your advantage, and I assure you that you will create connections with women that are more genuine and long-lasting.

I remember once when I had returned from a

trip to Paris, where I had gone to visit a friend, so I arrived at my home in Valencia, where at that time I was doing Airbnb to pay my rent. As soon as I walked in the door, I saw a girl getting ready in front of the mirror, in the room I had for rent. I was fascinated by her African beauty, her afro hair, her lovely face, and her light black skin. As soon as I saw her, I thought to myself: she has to be mine, I'm going to do it, I'm going to seduce her.

As a good host, I decided to introduce myself. I welcomed her to the city and proposed to her and her friend to meet up later that night. I remember planning to make some cocktails at my house with some friends, and they gladly accepted. They were happy to meet some local guys and enjoy some cocktails made by a professional bartender.

Night came. Lots of laughter. We all got to know each other, and after the Sex on the Beach cocktails, we decided to go dancing at Fox Congo, a pub near my house. We danced, we talked, and we had a great time. The night came to an end, and my roommate and I went back home; each of us slept in our own bed that night.

Since they were going to stay at my house for a week, we weren't in a hurry, so the next day we suggested going to the beach. It was summer, hence why we had so much free time... we went to the beach and spent the day there. When we returned home after getting ready, they felt like going out. My friends were tired and didn't want to do anything, but I really liked this girl and wanted to seduce her. Although I was tired too, I decided to push myself a bit. I acted as a guide and took them to some cool beach bars. For once, I had decided not to drink. (Yes, sometimes I can go out without drinking).

While we were sitting and talking, and I was having a Coca-Cola, I took advantage of her friend going to the bathroom, gathered my courage, and told her everything I thought about her. I told her that I liked her and found her very attractive. She laughed and asked me why I liked her, as she had noticed how I also looked at her friend. We both laughed, and I said, "Well... but you're the one I like the most, and that's why I'm telling you now and not your friend." I hadn't fully convinced her yet, so we continued enjoying ourselves until the place closed.

After closing, I suggested going for a swim at the beach. None of us had swimsuits, so we all swam half-naked. Once in the water, I looked into her eyes, she looked at me, and I kissed her without hesitation, to which she passionately returned the kiss. We got out of the water, but she still didn't fully trust me; she said she could tell I was a Playboy and that she wasn't going to spend the night with me. (The Playboy thing is true, I've never denied it).

That's when I discovered the theory I shared with you before about love. I told her, "Look, I like you, and we don't have to do anything tonight, but I would really like to sleep with you because I need a little love and companionship, and I don't want to spend the night alone." She laughed, agreed, and confessed to me that she didn't want to spend the night alone either and would love to sleep with me too, but emphasizing that we wouldn't do anything that night. I agreed to the deal.

We got to the house, and she agreed to sleep with me on the sofa bed in the living room. That night, all the rooms were rented out, and the house was full of guests. The funny thing is that in the end, she was the one who started touching me, and we ended up doing it. (This usually ends up happening). What's even funnier is that the next morning, the other guests, who were an older couple, saw us on the sofa in the living room. It was clear that something had happened that night. I definitely miss that apartment and everything that happened there with so many guests. If you have an apartment and live alone, I would recommend doing Airbnb; you'll earn some extra money, meet guests, and maybe even your future girlfriend.

In the end, we continued making plans for the week they stayed. My roommate ended up sleeping with her friend too, and I kept in touch with her.

In fact, she came to see me at my house again, this time without paying. We went on a trip together to Barcelona, and I also visited her a few times in Germany, specifically in Frankfurt.

We had a real connection, and although we've never been anything serious, to this day I still occasionally keep in touch with her, all because I played the card of love and companionship. After internalizing this principle of seduction in my subconscious, I confess that it has been much easier for me to seduce and create more genuine connections with the women I'm attracted to. Always with respect and naturalness, that's who I am, sensitive, romantic, I like to seduce, be liked, and be in good company. I don't see this as manipulation; I do it from the naturalness of my being. I emphasize this because taking advantage of this factor and creating false expectations in the other person will end up hurting them, and ultimately, that same harm you've done will come back to you like a boomerang.

If you feel that this is happening to you, and that maybe the other person is falling in love with you more than they should, it's advisable to talk to them about who you are, your feelings, and expectations to avoid misunderstandings and unnecessary headaches. This way, you'll be clear, and no one can accuse you of being manipulative, a jerk, or any other derogatory term. From my experience, in most cases, they accept my free-spirited nature, and we let things flow without any expectations.

SPEAK CLEARLY, WOMEN LOVE IT

CHAPTER XIV

Be very careful, you pervert, because I don't mean for you to go up to the girl and tell her you'd like to screw her right off the bat. Maybe it could work for you. Statistically speaking, you might have a one percent chance she says yes, at most two, being generous. But the most likely scenario would be her giving you a good slap, at best, and at worst, her filing a complaint and you spending a night in the slammer, in the company of law enforcement. Since I imagine that's not your plan, it's better not to speak so clearly and directly but to seek balance. I'll make it clearer for you later on.

Jokes aside, what I mean by this is that women like it when you tell them what you think and what your intentions are when the time comes. Because that's what a confident and self-assured man does: he expresses how he feels, as you already know... that's very attractive.

I'm telling you all this because I always observe men who are good at talking. They have no fear of starting a conversation with a stranger, but they never define things properly. They're often afraid to express what they really feel in that moment. They deceive themselves, thinking that expressing their feelings at that moment would be too aggressive or obscene on their part. The truth is, women love it when a man is sincere, speaks his mind, and reveals his intentions when the time comes. They don't want a man who hides his intentions and beats around the bush. From experience, I can tell you that by doing the latter, they'll get bored and go with someone else who does express themselves.

The reality is that this lack of clarity is why many men end up in the infamous "friend zone." They're not clear about their intentions, and women end up seeing them as just a friend for that very reason. So unless your goal is to make friends, express your intentions when the time comes.

To make it clear, I'm going to tell you the story of a very good friend, let's call him "Michael, the bad striker."

Michael is a guy who's good at talking to women, he makes them laugh, and you can tell they're having a good time. He has no problem stopping any stranger in a bar, on the street, or in any setting. In fact, he's quite good at creating interactions out of thin air. (Of which, sometimes, I take advantage as a good goal-scoring striker.)

I'm sure that if you saw him in action, you'd bet all your money on him leaving with the girl and being successful. Unfortunately, if you did, I assure you, you'd lose all your money. I don't mean to say that my friend never hooks up occasionally, but in most cases, he never does. He always wonders why, and no matter how much I tell him the reason, he doesn't want to understand. He tends to make excuses and thinks what he's doing is fine. That's why he's in the situation he's in. He's too proud to realize his mistakes.

Michael is like a bad striker in soccer that you don't want on your team; no matter how many crosses he gets, he never finishes, never scores, and ends up blaming others. This is because, no matter how good he is at talking to women and making them laugh, he never fully expresses what he really feels and what he would like to get out of that interaction. My friend is not clear, so he always ends up swinging through the jungle like Tarzan. Like a ship without a captain, he ends up adrift. Few women visit his bed for this reason.

Michael goes through this because he doesn't express what he wants. He's afraid of rejection and not confident enough. In fact, whenever I suggest he be clear about what he wants, that women love it when you tell them things as they are (because they rarely take the initiative), he always replies that he can't possibly say what he really thinks, that they'll think he's too forward, or in the worst-case scenario, a pervert. But those are just excuses he has in his head that prevent him from being a goal-scoring striker.

This is why my friend almost never ends up going home with the girl because he never expresses what he wants. For this reason, the woman usually gets bored of him because she knows what she's looking for, or at least she's waiting for someone to suggest something so she can have options and then decide what she wants. Generally, they end up going with another man who, unlike my buddy, knows what he wants.

So please, be clear always. Show what you think and what your intentions are. I'm not telling you to say it right at the beginning of the conversation, but do it once you see the signs that the woman is interested in you and enjoying your company. Once you've recognized these signs, take a chance and suggest going dancing, giving her a kiss, inviting her to your place, or all of the above.

I guarantee you, in most cases, if you've interpreted the signs correctly and the woman likes you, she'll accept almost anything you propose. And... in the worst-case scenario, you already know, you'll be rejected, you'll say goodbye politely, and life will go on as if nothing had happened.

Summing up everything said in this chapter, don't be like my friend Michael because that way, the only thing you'll achieve is not getting any-where. On the contrary, always have a pair of balls, be a wolf, and say what you think without fear. Express your ideas, your feelings, and intentions. By doing this, you'll realize how much women love a guy who is honest and sincere about what he thinks. As I've said a few times, women are usu-ally attracted to confident men who know what they want and are seeking. So by being clear, you'll indirectly demonstrate this to them, and if you've done your seduction job well, they'll be attracted to you. So please, do it for yourself and... BE CLEAR!

MEN AND WOMEN WANT TO HAVE FUN

CHAPTER XV

Sounds obvious, right? Who doesn't want to enjoy themselves and have a good time? You'd be surprised how many people have hired me for mentoring in seduction and personal development and yet don't grasp this obvious fact of life. It's astonishing to me. That's why I want to dedicate a chapter to this, to make it crystal clear and to dispel any mental cobwebs you may still have.

This ties in a lot with the previous chapter because understanding that women also want to have fun is a key factor that will help you speak clearly and express what you want. Knowing that they also want to have a good time. Internalizing this in your consciousness may help you the next time you want to speak frankly. Now, I'm not guaranteeing, my friend, that you'll always be successful when you express yourself. This is a game of probabilities, and having a clear understanding of the variables and factors in this seduction algorithm will help you emerge victorious and triumphant in more rounds.

I also want to debunk the idea you probably have in your head that women are fragile, pure, angelic beings who live in heaven and to whom you can't say anything sexual, dirty, or spicy. Dismissing your mythological myth, I'll tell you that nothing could be further from reality—women love sex just like you do. From my experience, I can assure you that I've met more than one who enjoys it even more than men.

I'm telling you all this so you can change your mental perspective. They generally have many suitors and are accustomed to being seduced. As you know, sex is part of this game. As a woman who has been seduced several times, I can guarantee you that probably any woman you want to seduce in the future will have more sexual experience than you. I can imagine this because you're reading this book. Don't let this intimidate you either; just accept it as a variable or possibility. You'll gain that experience later on.

Knowing all this, dear Casanova, we can safely assume that women love to be seduced by the right man and taken to bed. Of course, there are exceptions, but I'm speaking generally, based on what I've seen and experienced over these past few years. So, speaking in broad terms and now understanding that women, just like men, are dying for sex, dying to be seduced, desired, and to attract a man who can meet all those expectations. What's stopping you, the next time you're with a woman, from proposing to go somewhere else to have a good time? Surely she's more eager than you are, and she's probably been waiting for you to propose it already.

On the other hand, you may encounter a woman who doesn't want to move too fast, which is great too. Because if she decides to keep seeing you, at least she'll know your intentions, and if she agrees to keep seeing you, it's because she hopes you'll seduce her better to end up in bed with you.

In the worst case scenario, she'll tell you that you're not her type, and at least you'll stop wasting your time with her. Avoiding misunderstandings, wasting time, and unnecessary friend zones.

Assuming all this, let's acknowledge that there are nymphomaniacs in life, and many women who can't live without sex as much as a man. I know cases where a man has gone two, three, or even five years without sex, contacting me for help. They usually don't understand this knowledge that I'm sharing with you now. On the other hand, a woman who goes a year without sex is really rare. It happens, but generally they can't resist for more than a few months, and that's because they want to. After all, they have it easier because, generally, if they're moderately attractive, they'll always have some suitor waiting to get them into bed. And since they also love sex... why resist? The era of the insecure, inexperienced virgin maiden is over. Welcome to the 21st century where the princess has more sexual experience than the prince.

So, don't be intimidated, and let's learn from this. The other day when I was with the German girls (I imagine you'll remember them from some previous chapter), I came up with the idea to write this chapter. Let me tell you and set the scene.

As you know, they were on vacation, so as usual, they were looking to have a good time. The friend I had hooked up with the other night was talking to a guy she had met the same night I had gone out with them.

We were having drinks when this guy messaged her on her phone. He was pretty straightforward, even more so than I personally like. He wrote the following on WhatsApp or something like that:

"Hey gorgeous, how are you? I really wanted to get to know you better the other night. If you're up for it, I'm free after 10 p.m. I can pick you up in my car, and we can spend some time alone at the beach."

Surprisingly, she accepted. The funny thing is, the guy didn't speak English, but when it comes to the language of sex, you don't need words. I confess that this isn't my style, and I don't feel comfortable doing these kinds of things; I'm more romantic. But I'm telling you this to show you other examples of what happens and is also real, so you understand everyone's game.

Anyway, he came to pick her up at the bar where we were, so I was left with the friend. Since we all had to sleep together that night and we were in a caravan at a camping site a bit far from the city, I had to wait for the friend to come back and for my turn to have sex too.

I took a walk with the girl, we talked, and we spent a couple of hours waiting. Eventually, the other friend returned with the guy she had just slept with, with whom she communicated using Google Translate. As you can see, the girl knew what she wanted, and so did the guy. The other man arrived with the car, and like a good gentleman, he offered to drive the lady back to the campsite where they were staying. So, we all went together.

During the ride, I acted as an interpreter since he didn't speak English and she didn't speak Spanish. So, I found out that the man had four children, a girlfriend, and he had just cheated on her with the German girl, with the German girl knowing this whole story. The thing is, even knowing all that, she didn't mind going to have a good time with him at the beach.

As for me, I reflected on it, acknowledging that it wasn't my style in seduction at all, but in the end, it was another method. I found it intriguing, and that's why I want to share it with you now. So you're aware that both men and women ultimately want the same thing, and sometimes it's easier to be honest and say what it is than to beat around the bush.

As you may have noticed throughout the course of reading this book, each person is a different world, and a different approach to seduction must be applied to each individual. You're not going to flirt the same way with a twenty-year-old girl as you would with one in her thirties or forties. Nor would you approach someone from Asia the same as someone from South America or Europe. In seduction, it's always necessary to adapt to each scenario. But as you've also observed, there are common patterns that repeat themselves, regardless of whether you speak Swahili or Quechua. This pattern I'm discussing in this chapter is one of them, so internalize it, make it your own, and seize the opportunity the next time it presents itself. Forget about your mental blockages and understand that we're all looking to have a good time, so don't be afraid to suggest more enticing plans, to invite her to your house or your bed. You already know perfectly well that the worst thing that can happen is to be left with doubt.

WHAT DO I DO IF THE GIRL I LIKE IS WITH HER FRIENDS?

CHAPTER XVI

There's a great chance that the girl you're interested in isn't alone and is with her friends. I understand that this might be intimidating in some cases, and you might see it as a challenge. But hey, this is part of life, and you need to know how to handle such situations; otherwise, you might miss out on one of the best experiences of your life.

I see two possible scenarios here:

A) You've decided to go out on your own.
B) You have some moral support because you're with a friend.

Regardless of the scenario, there's always a right

way to act. Since both scenarios can happen, let's start with the first one to see what you can do if you find yourself in this situation.

Scenario A) The Lone Wolf

Let's say you've gone out alone. Perfect, that shows you've got guts and don't give a damn about going out solo. Now you've spotted that girl you're into, but she's with her friends, and you're not sure how to approach her. You feel embarrassed, intimidated, and you start overthinking it. The mental block kicks in. Your hands get sweaty, and you're nervous. But it's okay. You came to play, so let's play. Break the mental block. Get the courage to approach and talk to her.

In this scenario, the best thing you can do is first approach the girl you like and tell her why she caught your eye. She'll probably tell you she's with her friends and wants to hang out with them. Don't back off just yet, buddy. Now you'll have to talk to the friends and make a good impression on them. After talking to the girl you like, it's time to focus more on the friends. Your job is to earn their trust and respect while not forgetting about the girl you like.

Once you've gained the trust of everyone and see they're comfortable with you, it's time to turn your attention back to the girl you like. Suggesting going dancing is always a good idea because then you'll be the center of attention. This gives you the opportunity to move to the next step and try to kiss her or initiate more physical contact, like touching her hand or hip, and see how she responds. If you sense she's comfortable, you're in. If not, you'll have to assess the situation—whether she's playing hard to get or simply not interested.

In these kinds of solo scenarios, you'll need to put your social skills into practice more, as you'll need to grab everyone's attention while being alone. But once you get the hang of it, you'll realize it wasn't as hard as it seemed. Don't forget what you learned in the chapters on nonverbal communication and the art of conversation. They'll help you maintain the necessary standards to at least try to grab the group's attention, especially the girl you like. Remember, in life, nothing ventured, nothing gained.

Scenario B) The Wolf Goes with a Buddy or Buddies

The approach here is very similar to when you go solo. However, if you have the help of a friend, things are always easier. That is, as long as he's good at this whole flirting thing, or at least he's reading and trying to educate himself in seduction like you are. Otherwise, he'll be more of a burden. If your friend isn't good and is going to get in your way, I always think it's better to go it alone, but if you don't believe me, give it a shot. Maybe it'll happen that he's so bad that he makes you look like a Greek god of seduction in comparison, which could actually work in your favor.

Assuming you're both on the same level, in that case, one of you will have to break the ice and introduce yourselves to the group that caught your attention. There's no need to be too direct here. It's best if one person goes first and breaks the ice in a friendly manner without showing interest in any-one specific, and then invites the friend to join the group. Try to join as if you're a group of friends, as if you're looking to meet new people, which is ultimately what you're after. Bring up conversa-tion topics, and don't forget you'll have to involve everyone in the conversation (yes, even the fat one you're not interested in, you'll have to engage with her too). The objective, as always, is to gain the group's trust. Let them see you as easygoing, friendly, and eager to have a good time together.

This way, you'll create a more relaxed atmosphere since there won't be any overt displays of direct intentions, making communication and interaction more natural and advantageous for you if you know how to play your cards right.

Once you've achieved this, you should try to engage in individual conversations, each focusing on the girl who caught your attention the most. Don't fight over them; choose different girls for each of you. You also need to communicate with each other; otherwise, you'll end up fighting over the same girl, and neither of you will get her.

If you notice that both girls are receptive to you, do the typical thing—suggest dancing. If necessary, dance with the one you're not interested in to continue building trust within the group. Once you've gained the attention of the girl you like and you notice she's receptive, interested in you, and giving clear signs of positive nonverbal communication, it's time to be clear and take action. Hopefully, both of you will score, or just one. In the worst-case scenario, neither, but at least you'll have had a laugh and learned a bit more about relationships and social skills.

If you feel like it, I'll tell you another story. If not, skip the story and move on to the next chapter.

Morocco. Marrakech. Year 2018 or 2019. I don't remember well. I was around twenty-two or twenty-three years old. Now I'm almost twenty-seven or eight. The thing is, I was traveling in Morocco with a friend of mine.

The idea was to travel around for a month, which we more or less did. At that time, I wasn't the seducer I am now, but I wasn't the loser I was in London either. I was starting to see results in seduction, and it wasn't going too bad for me. But I still had a lot to learn. Let's say I was at an intermediate level. During that trip, I was obsessed with meeting a local woman, or two, to travel with them and my friend. In the end, from experience, I'll tell you that when you become obsessed with something, sooner or later you achieve it.

With this beautiful obsession, I found myself eating a delicious chicken tagine with my friend on the terrace of a restaurant. At the table next to us were two beautiful Moroccan women, with cinnamon skin, dark hair, big eyes, and a lovely smile. To add more excitement, they were sisters, which we realized later. I liked the younger one, and my friend liked the older one. So, we already knew which one each of us was going for.

I propose to my friend the plan I had in mind, and he confirms that he also felt attracted to them but that I had to make the first interaction since he didn't dare to do it. Giovanni Amato gets up. He visualizes his goal and approaches the table where those two beautiful women were, always with a good smile. I don't make any extravagant entrance,

I introduce myself, point to my friend, and say that we were interested in sitting with them, that we were looking to meet local people, and they seemed interesting to us. They accept and invite us to their table. (As you can see, I didn't go with any intention of flirting with them, at least that's what it seemed).

My friend comes with a big smile. (He couldn't believe what he had just achieved). I was also happy; I couldn't believe it had been so easy. We start introducing ourselves. We talk, ask them for recommendations for the trip, while showing interest in them, what they do with their lives, what they do for a living, and what they like to do in their free time. After chatting for a while and once we had gained some of their trust, we suggest that they show us around the city. They willingly accept, so we start sightseeing with them around the city. We end up having some very typical Moroccan mint teas at another terrace in the city. (Believe it or not, on that trip, I didn't drink alcohol, well maybe a beer or two, but we definitely had more tea than anything else). High on caffeine, it got dark, and each of us went back to our hotel, but not before exchanging contacts. I forgot to tell you that during the day, we had talked about making some plans together the next morning. (As I have mentioned before, sometimes it's very important to make small plans for the near future to see if there is interest, propose something different, and gain confidence).

The next morning, we had agreed to go on an excursion together to some nearby waterfalls, whose name I don't remember now. We spent a beautiful day with them in nature, getting to know each other better. We got ripped off with the taxis, the food, and everything, but in the end, they were delighted to have met us, and we were also delighted to have met them. Despite the typical scams you usually encounter in this country. But well, that's not a big problem. The important thing here is that we all had a good day and achieved the goal of gaining the trust of the two sisters.

When night fell and we were back in the city, my friend went with the sister to a nightclub in the city, while I stayed with the other one, taking a walk and getting to know the city at night. As we walked, I confessed to her that I liked her and wanted something more with her. She said she felt the same way, but in that country, we couldn't go anywhere together unless we were married, as it was punishable by law, even with jail time. Things in Muslim countries. Since I didn't believe it, I took her to the place where we were staying, and indeed, they didn't let me spend the night with her, but at least I didn't end up in jail for trying.

Since the girl was also eager, we ended up getting up to some mischief here and there in the streets, in the alleys of the medina, under the moonlight. Luckily, no one saw anything, as I think it could have gotten me into big trouble.

I returned to the hotel with my friend, with a big smile, satisfied with what had just happened. Of course, I told him the story while he was dying of envy because he hadn't done anything with the other sister yet; he hadn't even dared to tell the girl he was attracted to her. Something he would do later, following my advice.

Fortunately, the younger sister had liked me quite a bit, so after resuming the journey with my friend and visiting several cities, we met the two sisters again. This time we went to visit them in their hometown, Ouarzazate, with the intention of picking them up there and all going on a trip to the desert together.

With quite a bit of discretion, we took the bus. They sat in the front seat, and we sat in the back, as they didn't want their father to find out that they were going to go with two tourists to the desert for a night. As you may know, or if not, I'll tell you now, in those kinds of Muslim countries, it's not well seen for two women to travel with guys they just met a few weeks ago. The good thing was that this fact added a lot more excitement to the story, although we received some disapproving looks from the local population.

In the desert, we had a great time. We walked through the dunes, rode camels, and drank more tea. As night fell, we went to sleep in the tents, after having a drum concert in the camp, along with a typical dinner from the area near the fire. Since there weren't as many rules in the desert, we were able to spend the night with the two sisters, my friend in one tent and me in the next. We could hear everything because the tents were close, so it was quite funny; the sisters spoke in Arabic among themselves, seemingly surprised by what each one was doing, especially the older one of the two. There were lots of laughs.

On the return journey, I must confess that I cried because I had grown very fond of this affectionate and attractive girl, so it was a bit sad. She cried too, and after spending the last hours together in the taxi back, we had to say goodbye, but not before she gave me a little gift for the journey back to our destination. (As I've told you before, I'm a romantic, what more can I say…).

I kept in touch with her for about a year through chat; we always talked about seeing each other again, but unfortunately, it never happened. Even today, sometimes I think of her and smile at all the experiences we had on that trip. That's life. The point here is that if I hadn't had the guts to get up and talk to them in the restaurant where we met, none of this would have happened, and I wouldn't have had such a beautiful trip with my friend and the two lovely sisters.

So you see, if you carry out seduction well, it will

always give you memories to reminisce, stories to tell, and very positive life experiences. Meeting interesting people, maintaining friendships, and having a great time, all wrapped up in one.

AWAKEN HER SEXUAL DESIRE

CHAPTER XVII

By now, you've learned to recognize the subtle gestures indicating that a woman is attracted to you, as well as how to start a conversation, overcome mental blocks, and a few other tricks. I hope all of this has become clear to you, so now I'll address a very important topic: "How to generate sexual tension and awaken sexual desire."

Let's suppose that your date has gone great. You've been talking, there's mutual interest, and everything is flowing smoothly. But of course, you're wondering: "How do I get her into bed?" Perfect. For that, it's essential to awaken her sexual desire and create the famous sexual tension we've all heard of at some point. But... you may be wondering, how do you do this? I'll try to explain it to you next.

Let's consider another example: you're sitting in a bar, getting to know that woman you've been longing to have a date with. You're conversing smoothly, she looks into your eyes and you into hers, sparks begin to fly. She smiles at you, and you smile back. A strong desire to kiss her starts to build up in your mind, probably in hers too, but you hesitate out of fear of making a fool of yourself, and you end up getting blocked. Luckily, you've already learned how to overcome mental blocks, as well as the fact that women love honesty and clarity. You gather the courage to touch her hand; you notice that she likes it and she caresses your fingers. You start to feel nervous, but this is a good sign, so there's no need to panic. You move closer to her, and you notice that she's comfortable with your presence, she's not uncomfortable; on the contrary, she becomes nervous too. You start to gaze at her lips, and she realizes it, starting to bite them and run her fingers over them, showing that she likes you looking at her lips and is probably expecting something more from you.

In this situation, it's your turn to act. You can kiss her; you can take the leap, or if you're feeling intimidated, you can directly ask for it in a witty way. I usually use this line: "I'm sorry, but I can't continue this conversation; your lips are distracting me, and I can't keep talking to you unless I give you a kiss." This usually works for me, but it would be best if you didn't copy me and found your own. However, if you're feeling stuck, maybe copying me could work. Nevertheless, as you may have noticed, I always recommend using your own phrases, which will come to you with practice.

Let's suppose it worked, and she gave you that kiss. In this case, congratulations, you've successfully awakened her sexual desire. So, you can relax a bit, continue talking to her while gazing into her eyes and lips, which will further pique her interest and heighten sexual tension. You'll continue kissing her occasionally, always being the one to break the kiss to maintain the sexual tension intensely.

You're doing great; she's loving your kisses and wants more, but you're rationing them because your goal is to keep that sexual tension at its peak. (Let me explain this briefly: when you're the one to break the kiss, you typically make the other person want more, but this way, you'll be the one controlling the sexual tension, allowing you to handle the situation better. Also, rationing the kisses will make her want more. You can't be kissing her all the time, or she'll get tired, and she'll be the one to end the kiss, putting you under her sexual influence. So, it's best to be the one in control).

Resuming, you're maintaining the sexual tension at its peak, passionately talking, occasionally kissing her and taking sips of your drink. You can maintain this situation for as long as you want, but here's a suggestion: when you feel the sexual tension reaching its limit, it's time to suggest going somewhere more private. You'll need to suggest going to your place, hers, or a hotel, whichever you prefer.

If you've played your cards right, she'll usually accept without any issues, and you'll end up in bed with her. It could also happen that the woman doesn't want to move so fast, which often occurs. In that case, no worries; continue as before and try to have a good time with her. She'll probably come around on the second or third date. She'll also know what your intentions are, so if she decides to keep seeing you, she'll know what will eventually happen. Don't forget that this is also positive.

So, in these situations, I think the most important thing is to break the ice by giving a kiss. Let's say the kiss is always the first step to awaken that sexual tension or connection. Once that's done, if you do your job well in seduction, you'll generally end up in bed with her, as it indicates that she's sexually attracted to you because if she wasn't, she would have never accepted a kiss from you. (As always, there are exceptions, but try to stick with this idea).

To make it clearer, I'll provide you with a step-by-step guide for awakening her sexual desire and gradually increasing sexual tension. I think it'll be a more intuitive way to reinforce what you've learned. Plus, you can review it whenever you want.

Guide to Awakening Her Sexual Desire and Creating a Connection.

· Preliminaries:

Before you start, it's crucial to ensure there's an emotional connection and mutual consent. The key is open communication and reading the signs, as you've learned in previous chapters.

· Step 1: **Passionate Gazes** (Public Setting):

Begin with eye contact and smiles. When you meet her eyes, hold the gaze for a second longer than usual to create a special connection. Look into her eyes and then to her lips, repeating this process. This will generate more tension.

· Step 2: **Seek Subtle Contact** (Ensuring Comfort):

During conversation, lightly touch her arm or hand while sharing something funny. This light physical contact will establish a more intimate connection. Also, it ensures she feels comfortable with you. If she doesn't withdraw her hand, arm, or leg, it's a good sign, so you can proceed to the next step.

· Step 3: **Seduction Game** (Creating a Playful Atmosphere):

Introduce slightly daring comments into the conversation to create a playful and complicit atmosphere. Use humor and emotional intelligence to read her reactions. You can compliment her lips, the color of her hair, her beautiful eyes, or whatever you find attractive about her. This subtly demonstrates your intentions and increases tension, which is your goal.

• Step 4: **Kiss Time** (Transition to Desire):

When you feel the tension has increased, move in for a passionate kiss. Start gently and assess her response. Kisses are key to intensifying the connection. Remember what I discussed in previous pages. If you don't feel comfortable taking the leap, you can always ask for it in a witty way.

• Step 5: **Transition to an Intimate Environment** (Private Setting):

Invite her to a more private place. This can be your house or a quiet place where you can be alone. The transition creates a more conducive environment for intimacy. Remember that she may not want to move so fast; in that case, you'll stay in this step and continue with the next on another date. Sometimes, things don't go as planned, no matter how well the date went.

• Step 6: **Explore Her Body More Intimately** (Awaken Physical Desire):

As the interaction becomes more intimate, gently explore her body with touches and caresses. Gradual tactile exploration will increase physical desire. You can touch her legs, arms, buttocks, breasts, but not the pussy yet, tiger. This will stimulate her desire.

• Step 7: **Constant Communication** (Pay Attention to Signals):

Communication is essential at every step. Make sure both of you are comfortable and willing to move forward. Ask and listen, making sure to respect boundaries. By this, I mean avoiding uncomfortable situations and respecting the other person. As you know, each person is different, and what worked with one might not work with another. For example, one may like it when you touch her breasts, but another may feel uncomfortable in a public place. Simply communicate and pay attention to signals. Your goal is not to end up in jail.

• Step 8: **Intensification of Kisses** (Heading to Bed):

You're already at a house or hotel. Intensify kisses and caresses as the moment approaches. Create an atmosphere of shared desire that prepares the ground for the next step. Here, the idea is to further awaken sexual desire to seek physical pleasure. Now you can touch her pussy, champ.

• Step 9: **Intimate Moment** (Bed Entry):

When both are ready, transition naturally to the bed. This step should feel smooth and consensual. Comfort and trust are key. Let's say things are a bit cold; you can always have a drink to relax the atmosphere. The important thing here is not to force anything and let both of you feel the desire to go to bed; usually, it will be noticeable and natural.

• Step 10: **Enjoyment Time** (Your Moment):

Here, I can't tell you anything else, tiger; you'll have to do the work. As advice, you could have talked before this interaction about what you both like in bed, so there are no surprises. However, this isn't necessary from my point of view, although it can help. (I've done it before). Try to make her come, as this will surely lead to another date if you're up for it. Don't get nervous and try to enjoy yourselves.

Let me tell you a personal story to make all of this very clear and leave no doubts. About a month ago, I had a date with a girl I met on a dating app, specifically Bumble. She was a Venezuelan girl, a bit tanned, and quite cute. The thing is, while chatting with her on WhatsApp, she asked me the typical question about what I was looking for on the app. She emphasized that she wasn't looking for sex and just wanted to meet people. I thought it was a good approach and accepted the deal. (Sometimes they just do this to weed out perverts who only want sex without any prior interaction).

We agreed to meet at a small shopping center that was halfway between our respective homes.

We met, introduced ourselves, and decided to go grab a drink at a nearby bar. I was pretty relaxed because in the end, I was just going to meet her and see how things went; I wasn't looking for anything specific. I didn't have much to do that afternoon, so it was the best plan available.

Some things I can't help but do automatically, I found myself staring into her eyes, occasionally glancing at her lips, which were quite full and caught my attention. Honestly, I was just talking normally and had no intention of seducing her (well, maybe I did, sometimes I like to be liked and to seduce just for the sake of it).

The thing is, without me saying anything, she started to embarrass me a bit, telling me that my gaze was very intense, and even though I had a "good boy" face, it was obvious that I was a fuck-boy and a seducer. She was sure that I went out with many women. There was a phrase she said that stuck with me, which might be true. I quote verbatim: "You know, from my experience, I've learned that those who talk the most about having sex, act cocky, and brag are the ones who have sex the least and usually are losers, whereas you, you seem relaxed, you have a good guy look, you seem confident, and you have a very intense gaze, so I imagine you must be a seducer, because those who act good are the worst." (She wasn't wrong). I responded with a laugh, saying that none of that was true, that I was shy and a geek.

As you can see, the girl had me figured out perfectly, but sometimes, and often, that ends up attracting even more attention because they see you as a confident guy who knows what he wants and attracts women, so she ends up wanting to unravel what makes you so special and desired by other women. That's more or less what happened in this case and in many others because in the end, I always try to be honest and lead with my natural self.

Resuming the story, after she let all of that out, the bar was closing, and we moved to another one, specifically to "100 Montaditos." It was Wednesday, which meant there was an offer, so we took advantage of it for a cheap dinner.

I was sitting across from her, and I kept looking at her, as I usually do with any woman, but she kept getting uncomfortable, telling me to stop looking at her like that because my gaze made her nervous. All of this made me laugh, so I looked at her even more intensely, looked her in the eyes, winked at her, and occasionally touched her hand to create sexual tension and confirm whether I was right or not.

Obviously, all of this had its results, so I politely asked her to come closer to me, which she did. While we continued talking and looking into each other's eyes, I took the opportunity to put my hand on her leg, and indeed, she became even more nervous. She was eager for me to kiss her, but I wasn't going to give her that reward just yet. So, I focused on creating even more sexual tension, continuing with the looks, caresses, and playful smiles. Meanwhile, we continued with a slightly hotter conversation, talking about previous sexual experiences and what we liked to do in bed

In the end, I decided to kiss her, which she eagerly welcomed. I played a bit with her, as I mentioned earlier, kissing her, stopping, and continuing to caress her to further arouse her desire. The thing is, she ended up asking me about the size of my cock, to which I said she could feel it herself, so I put my hand there while continuing to kiss her, and things were getting heated. I won't delve into more explicit details because this isn't an erotic book, but I'm sure you get the idea.

Ultimately, I suggested going to a more intimate place, in this case, it had to be her place since I'm currently back at my parents' house. (A bit of a drag, but it's temporary, and I'm still getting laid anyway). Surprisingly, she declined my invitation, saying she didn't feel like moving so fast because, according to her, she didn't sleep with just anyone. I insisted a bit more, she rejected me again, so I left her alone, and after a while, we said goodbye with a kiss, and each went home.

We met again, where there was the same sexual tension I mentioned before, more kisses, and even more touching, but she still didn't want me to go to her place. I hope that the third date will be the charm.

As you can see in this story, there was clearly a very strong sexual tension between us, in fact, I was surprised because I've been with women with less sexual tension whom I ended up going to bed with. That's why I insist here that every person is different, and sometimes, as in this case, no matter how much tension there was, it didn't mean it would end up in bed with her. But hey, in the end, I had a great time and lots of laughs, and I hope there will be a third date where it does end up in bed with her.

Nevertheless, as I've told you many times, seduction is not a robotic and mathematical algorithm, there are many variables and factors that can turn what seemed like a clear triumph into a failure and vice versa, so you always have to be attentive and open to a possible unexpected change of course.

I hope this chapter has served you well, and you have learned from both the theory and the personal story. As for me, I bid you farewell, I'll stop writing for today, I'm going to have a beer with a friend, and then most likely meet up with a friend tonight.

BREAK FREE: TAKE CONTROL OF YOUR SOCIAL CIRCLE

CHAPTER XVIII

In this chapter, I want to focus on the hypothetical scenario (which happens quite often) where you find yourself in a group setting, but the group isn't on the same page as you and doesn't want to play along. Let's suppose you're with a group of friends, but you're in the mood to flirt while they're not interested, maybe because they have girlfriends or simply aren't feeling it. But you're eager to meet new people and refuse to be swayed by the group's dynamics because you've learned that following the herd is what sheep do. Hopefully, you've already decided not to be one of them.

I understand that this situation can sometimes

be a bit of a drag since you're up for it but the rest of the group isn't, which can demotivate you and make you stop flirting due to peer pressure. However, I believe that would be a mistake. I'm telling you this because it's a scenario I've personally experienced, and I think it can happen to anyone, and sometimes it's frustrating to find yourself in that situation.

So, how can this be resolved? Very simple. Either you break away on your own and do your thing, which isn't a bad option and is self-explanatory as I've already provided examples of how to act solo before. Or, on the contrary, you take advantage of being in a group and try to integrate other people, leveraging the group's comfort in your favor. By doing this, you'll come across as a friendly and outgoing guy who enjoys meeting new people and having fun, which will make others notice you in a positive light. Additionally, indirectly, you'll also build more trust with the other people because being in a social environment and having your own group always helps ease tensions, thereby creating a sort of false confidence in the other group or person you're trying to integrate.

This is due to the simple nature of human beings, as we must not forget that we are social beings, and generally, we love being in the company of pleasant and friendly people. Therefore, taking advantage of this for seduction is undoubtedly a good strategy and a good idea to consider when you find yourself in a similar situation. This way, you'll be prepared to use the group you're in to your advantage and capture the attention of that person who caught your eye at first sight.

Let me give you an example to make this clearer. A few years ago, when I was traveling solo in Thailand, I was meeting up that night with a group of very friendly German couples I had met that same day at the hostel. I was the only single one among them, and therefore the only one interested in flirting and meeting new people. As you can imagine, that idea didn't even cross their minds, as they were quite content with their respective partners.

We were having drinks at a Thai bar while playing the famous UNO board game. We were having a great time, chatting about our travels, adventures, and life in general. As you might guess, there came a moment when I was more interested in meeting new people and socializing with new folks (or rather, I was in the mood for seducing). So, I took advantage of the social situation I was in to steer it towards what I wanted, in this case, a beautiful Thai woman. (This is what seducers usually do: capitalize on the environment and opportunities that life presents to lead them to their territory).

As fate would have it, right next to our table, there was a small group of about three Thai women, chatting among themselves while sipping cocktails. I immediately noticed that they glanced at us from time to time, as we were laughing, talking loudly, and drawing a bit of attention in the bar. So, I used the environment and the game we were playing to invite the other group to join us in playing Uno. Obviously, the people I was with thought it was great that I integrated new members, and the women also thought it was great to become part of the group. After all, almost everyone enjoys socializing, especially if you approach in a friendly and amicable manner. Frankly, it would have been quite odd for them to reject the proposal.

So, we pushed the tables together, and the two groups found ourselves playing and sharing experiences. I wasn't really looking to flirt at all; on the contrary, I was quite relaxed and happy to be sharing that moment with everyone. So, indirectly, I was attracting quite a bit of attention because I was the one who had brought the groups together, and we were all laughing. Also, being relaxed, friendly, and true to myself indirectly made the group trust me more because I was being easygoing, fun, natural, and spontaneous.

We played several rounds, and after finishing the game, we focused on getting to know each other better. As usual, there was a girl who caught my attention, so I became more interested in her, seeking more individual conversations to get to know each other better and try to capture her attention even more. My goal was to seduce her, which I was doing quite effectively. As we continued talking, everyone participated in the group conversation, and we shared anecdotes among ourselves.

Suddenly, a song I liked started playing, so I took that opportunity to invite the Thai girl who had caught my eye to dance. Being in a relaxed and group setting, she accepted without any problem. I also emphasize that by inviting her to dance, I was showing that I was truly interested in her. So, indirectly, I was following the steps I mentioned in the previous chapter to arouse her desire.

As we danced, we gazed into each other's eyes, both smiling, touching hands, and there was physical contact. In short, it was clear that there was chemistry and tension between us, so I kissed her affectionately, and she returned the kiss. We danced a little more, sharing a few more kisses accompanied by caresses, and then rejoined the group. We all stayed together for another hour or so until it got later, and everyone wanted to go home.

At that moment, I seized the opportunity to speak privately with the Thai girl I liked and suggested going to a more intimate place, which was the hotel where I was staying at the time in Bangkok. She enthusiastically accepted my invitation, and we spent a lovely night together.

The next morning, we went out for lunch, and she showed me around the city, which is always great when guided by a local who knows where to take you. In the end, I met up with her a few more times, but I had to say goodbye to her as I had to continue my solo journey. I could have stayed longer, but I preferred to continue on my way to my next destination, which was another city a little further north, specifically Pai. In that city, I would meet new people again, but that's another story.

As you may have noticed, these situations are a great opportunity to flirt and meet new people. Ultimately, as human beings, being in a group and being sociable with another group tends to transmit good vibes and relax the atmosphere. This indirectly conveys that you're not seeking anything sexual, but rather just looking to socialize, meet new people, and be friendly. As a result, you'll create a relaxed environment, get to know the other people within the comfort of your group, and most likely, catch someone's attention simply by initiating the first interaction. Additionally, the game of seduction becomes easier as none of your friends will be competing with you since they're not in the mood to flirt for whatever reason, whether they have a partner like in this case or for any other reason. So, it would be a good scenario for you to take advantage of and possibly end up flirting that night.

Keep in mind, this is just an example from a few years ago that I wanted to share with you. To apply it, you don't have to be the only one interested in flirting; it could also work if you're with a group of friends who are in the same vibe as you, and it could yield similar results. This is just an idea that might come in handy when you find yourself in a similar situation and feel like merging groups. So, remember, relax, be yourself, and always try to have fun. This is usually the most attractive and attention-grabbing approach, which will make the task of seduction easier for you.

FLIRTING MASTERY: YOUR ULTIMATE GUIDE

CHAPTER XIX

In this chapter, I will discuss a series of techniques or strategies that I have developed over the years, based on my experience in the field of seduction. They are not really techniques or strategies, but rather situations that can arise in everyday life and that can be exploited to flirt and achieve your goal of seducing that person who caught your attention. That's why I think it's a good idea to share them with you, because I'm sure that, at some point, you will find yourself in a similar situation and this could help you. So... Let's get started!

The Anaconda Technique.

Let me set the scene for you: the anaconda is an animal that is heavy and large, so it can't hunt and catch its prey by surprise. If it did, its size would give it away, causing its prey to flee and leaving it hungry. Instead, its strategy for getting food is quite simple. It hides in a place where there is water, capable of going for days without eating, knowing that sooner or later, an animal will come to drink there. So, it waits for its prey, hidden in the water, relaxed, calm, without drawing attention to itself. Pity the poor little animal that goes to drink there, unaware of the lurking serpent. While the animal drinks, the anaconda seizes the opportunity, emerges from its hiding place, and... gets itself a good meal. It will then move and find another hiding spot to repeat the same strategy. As you can see, it's a strategy with quite a bit of cunning.

You might say, "You're crazy! That's the animal world!" But... what does this have to do with seduction? Let me explain.

In essence, it's about being in the right place at the right time. Let's say you're reading a book in a park, and suddenly an attractive woman walks by and catches your eye. You can act like the anaconda and take the opportunity to get to know her, or you can let it pass and regret it later. Let's consider another scenario: you've decided to go out alone for the night. You're having a drink at a bar or on the street, wherever you prefer, when suddenly a group of people sits down next to you, catching your attention. Once again, it's up to you whether to act or not. Let's try another scenario:

you're at a nightclub. Alone. A bit nervous, but you're keeping it cool. You take a sip of your favorite drink. Suddenly, a song you like starts playing. You start dancing and look around. You notice a beautiful woman looking at you. You lock eyes with her. She smiles at you, and... once again, the choice is yours. Will you act and talk to her? Or will you watch as someone else takes her away? If you decide to act in any scenario I've described, I call this the Anaconda Technique.

Translated to human terms, it's about seizing the opportunities life gives you to meet people, being in the right place at the right time. You could say it's a technique because, if you're observant, you can anticipate where people might show up. Maybe it's the main square in your city, the trendiest bar, the central park, the beach, the lake, an airport, public transportation, or any other setting. The point is, you can go solo to the environment you choose, be yourself, and use this technique inspired by the famous anaconda to your advantage. Not only will you build confidence by putting yourself in uncomfortable situations by going solo, but you'll also develop your social skills better and have a great opportunity to meet new and unique people.

This one is more intuitive, but I'll explain it anyway. Imagine you're out with a friend, you've danced, had a good time, and met a group of interesting girls, but unfortunately, they had to leave early. Suddenly, you glance at the clock and realize that the club you're in is about to close soon. You start to feel nervous, thinking you'll end up going home alone, which isn't very appealing. Don't worry, this is where the "door technique" comes in, the famous age-old strategy.

As you may have noticed, when the party ends, there's always a group of people lingering outside, chatting, waiting for a new plan to emerge, killing time, or simply sobering up a bit. This could be your moment to get what you've been looking for all night.

Coincidentally, there's a group of two girls who just stepped out the door, lighting up a cigarette and chatting away. You're with your friend, having a relaxed conversation, finishing off that last drink you had.

What would you do? Would you go talk to them, intending to propose a new plan or just get to know them? Or... would you stand there silently? Personally, I'd go for the first option, but that's up to you.

I call this funny little mental game the "door

technique". Occasionally, it works because if we think psychologically and analyze human behavior, when the party ends, many people are left wanting to do something else, whether it's fueled by alcohol, drugs, or just enthusiasm. So, if you're smart and observant enough, you can approach that group that caught your eye, suggest an alternative plan, strike up a conversation to get to know each other, and head somewhere else. You could suggest going to another bar, nightclub, that after-party you know about, or suggest having drinks at someone's house. If it goes well, you might end up hooking up that night. If it doesn't, at least you'll have had a good laugh. In the end, you have nothing to lose, and a lot to gain if it goes well. So, give it a try next time you're out. Remember the courtyard technique.

The Jumping Spider Technique

Let me set the scene for you. The other day, I was watching a documentary on Netflix about animals. Sometimes, I enjoy watching animal documentaries because I believe there are many behaviors in the animal kingdom that are applicable to humans. After all, we're all animals, albeit more evolved, but we all come from the same world. Therefore, there are behaviors or patterns that are similar in both humans and animals, or in this case, arthropods.

As I was saying... This spider is a very interesting and colorful one. It's quite small in size but has very striking colors in the male, while the female is more grayish in color. When mating season arrives, it's the male's job to catch the attention of the female. (Just like humans in most cases... what a coincidence...)

To catch the attention of his future mate, the male spider performs a curious and peculiar dance, worth seeing, performing acrobatics, jumps, and showing off his beautiful colors. The female, on the other hand, watches, analyzes, and chooses the male with the best dance and who captures her attention the most. Beware of the male who approaches without her consent, as this spider tends to eat them if she doesn't choose them. Quite dangerous. Luckily, we don't have the same fate. At most, and in the worst-case scenario, we might get rejected, which isn't a big problem compared to this spider.

As you can see, translated into us human beings, and specifically men, it's about knowing how to dress, how to move, how to look elegant, how to appear more confident, how to act. In short, it's about standing out from the rest. It could be your charm, your wit, your appearance, your ingenuity, your intelligence, or any characteristic you can think of, or all of the above. So, you have to discover yours and make them stand out. The key is, in some way, you have to grab attention because if you don't, you'll be lucky... because at least you won't end up as dinner, but you'll still be alone, and nobody likes to be alone.

The Technique of the Friend of the One Who Is Seeing Your Friend

This is more of a piece of advice in case you hadn't thought about it. Let me set the scene for you. Imagine one of your friends met a girl the other day when you went out together, and he's already been on a couple of dates with her. Maybe it would be a good idea to suggest to your friend that he should think about you and propose to his date to hang out with one of her friends as well. This way, you'll find yourself in a friendly scenario with your friend, his fling, maybe a couple of your other friends, and the new friends.

This is a very good way to flirt and meet new people because when your friend is seeing that girl, bringing her friends along can be a great idea. The atmosphere will be more relaxed, there won't be as much pressure, and more or less, the friend will have an idea of what's going on.

This may sound trivial, but it's a very good leveraging technique because, like in trading, here you'll be leveraging your friend's friend to arrange a double date.

You can also apply this in reverse and be the generous friend who sets up a date for that guy you know who struggles to meet women.

The Street Approach Technique

This technique is somewhat related to the anaconda technique but has some slight differences. As the name suggests, it involves being out on the street.

You can apply this technique either alone or with a friend. It's quite simple: just be out on the street. Let's say there's a neighborhood near where you live where people tend to spend time outside, walking around, having a drink, and sharing moments.

In this case, as a good seducer that you've decided to become, you would just go about your business and try to initiate social interactions from scratch. In addition to the possibility of meeting someone interesting, you'll also have the opportunity to practice your social skills and gain experience in this field.

So, the next time you're bored at home, head out onto the street, go to an area where you know there's some street activity in the city, and dare to talk to strangers. It's up to you whether you want to go alone or with someone else. But from my point of view, it wouldn't hurt to go alone sometimes because that way you'll gain confidence, self-assurance, and you'll also put your social skills to the test.

The LGBTQ Club Technique

"But Giovanni, what are you saying?" If you heard me correctly, I said LGBTQ club. Let me explain.

First, if you're clear about your sexuality, you shouldn't mind being in this type of club, as your goal won't be to flirt with a man.

Second, I'm sharing this with you based on personal experience. It's not a secret, but perhaps you weren't aware of it. I mean, it's entirely possible to flirt with a woman in an LGBTQ club, and sometimes it even makes the task easier.

You might be wondering why. It's quite simple. In an LGBTQ club, women generally feel more relaxed because they know nobody will hit on them since most of the men there aren't interested in relationships with women. Therefore, they're generally more receptive to striking up a conversation with you.

This works in your favor because, in addition to wondering why a heterosexual guy is there, she might also see you as someone with a more open mindset, unconcerned about social categorizations, and displaying self-assurance. As you've learned in this book, this attracts and generates curiosity.

So, if you play your cards right, this can be a great scenario to meet and seduce a woman. Personally, every time I've been to this type of club, I've ended up flirting for all the reasons I've mentioned. In fact, the last time was just a few days ago on a trip to London before finishing this chapter. The girl even told me she hadn't expected to flirt in a place like that. She had gone there to avoid being hit on by men, but I had been different, and she was attracted to me. As an anecdote, I met her on Friday and was seeing her until I left London the following Tuesday. Perhaps I'll tell the whole story later, in another book.

Try going to an LGBTQ club one day and see what happens. Just remember, you'll have to talk to women; otherwise, nothing will happen, or maybe a guy will hit on you, boosting your self-esteem and ego – after all, everyone likes to be liked. So, go ahead and see what happens.

SEDUCTION IN EVERYDAY LIFE

CHAPTER XX

Now that you're reaching the end, I can call you a Master Seducer. So, master, you just need one final push to earn your seduction mastery. This is about integrating seduction into your everyday life, not just to seduce a woman, but for any aspect of daily life.

Let me explain further. Seduction is an art, a science. It's about getting what you want and what you think is most beneficial for you from any situation you can imagine. You can use it to flirt, to close a deal, to convince your friend to take a trip, to show confidence in a job interview, or simply to be perceived as someone confident and charismatic.

With all this in mind, let me summarize how seduction can be used in each area of everyday life.

Social Seduction: Connecting Naturally

Social seduction involves the ability to build authentic connections with people in your everyday environment, whether at social events, family gatherings, or casual outings. It's about picking up on the body language of those around you, conducting a superficial analysis of each person so that you can position yourself better, anticipate people's movements, and always aim to earn the respect of others while benefiting from the group. The goal is to get to know people and understand how they may interact with you, what you can expect from them, and what you can offer them. Ultimately, the objective is to come out on top and prevent anyone from taking advantage of you.

Some key principles include:

•**Openness and Authenticity**: Being natural in your interactions, showing genuine interest in others. This will make you perceived as someone of high value, thus earning respect, and people will be more open to helping you.

•**Empathy and Active Listening**: Understanding others' emotions, showing that you care about what they say, while also expressing your own opinion and point of view without being swayed by others.

•**Nonverbal Communication**: Using positive body language that conveys confidence and openness. Also, analyzing the body language of others to understand their position.

Practical Example: Imagine you're at a party. Instead of focusing on impressing others, you decide to listen to them and share authentic stories about yourself. This creates genuine and lasting connections while also attracting more attention.

Exercise: Choose an upcoming social event. Focus on listening to others and sharing authentic stories about yourself.

Goal: Build more genuine and authentic connections.

Seduction in the workplace isn't about manipulation but about showcasing your skills and personality in a way that makes you memorable and respected in the professional environment. The goal is to be perceived as someone confident, trustworthy, and decisive, making others admire and respect you, which indirectly facilitates your work.

Key principles include:

•**Assertive Communication**: Express your ideas clearly and confidently, not being swayed by others' opinions. Set boundaries to earn respect. Also, listen to and respect others' opinions.

•**Professional Empathy**: Understand your colleagues' and bosses' perspectives. Similarly, express your views respectfully, even if they differ from your coworkers'. This conveys respect and trust, making your colleagues value and respect you more.

•**Impactful Presentation**: Stand out not only for your work but also for how you present it. Learn the names of all your colleagues. Talk to them. Ask about their lives, their weekends. Showing this small interest will make your coworkers hold you in high esteem and respect.

Practical Example: In a meeting, carefully choose

your words to express your ideas clearly and effectively. This not only makes you stand out but also builds a reputation as an effective communicator.

Exercise: Show interest in those around you at work, starting by learning everyone's names, asking about their day-to-day, showing genuine interest, and generally being friendly, approachable, and enjoyable to be around.

Goal: Stand out not only for your work but also for how you interact with others.

Sales Seduction: Persuasion with Customer Focus

Sales seduction involves understanding the needs of the customer, persuading them ethically, and offering your service or product. It's about building social relationships and showing genuine interest in your potential customers.

Key principles include:

•**Customer Empathy**: Understand their concerns and needs. The more you know about the customer, the easier it will be to make a sale. This can be as simple as genuinely caring about them. Learn their name, ask about their family, their job situation; in short, show genuine and natural curiosity about them. The goal is to make them feel comfortable with you, so you can sell to them effectively.

•**Persuasive Language**: Use words and tones that resonate with the customer. You need to know what they like, how they speak, and how they express themselves. By adapting to their language and preferences, you'll connect with them, making the sale easier. This isn't manipulation but seduction.

•**Win-Win Negotiation**: Seek solutions that benefit both the customer and you. This principle can be applied to any aspect of life.

Practical Example: Imagine you work in sales.

When approaching a customer, focus on understanding their needs before presenting your product. This not only closes sales but also builds long-term relationships.

Exercise: Imagine being a potential customer for your own product or service. Identify their concerns and needs. Analyze how you can address their needs with the product you offer.

Goal: Adjust your sales approach to address those concerns.

<u>**Seduction in Everyday Life:
Transforming Common Situations**</u>

Seduction in everyday life involves applying seductive principles in your daily routine to enhance interactions and common situations. It can be when you go shopping, when you exercise, when you travel, or any everyday situation you can think of.

Key principles include:

·Positive Communication: Conveying messages in an optimistic manner. Radiating positive energy at all times is a key principle to ensure that people around you perceive you as a joyful person whom they can trust and who spreads positivity. Achieving this makes people esteem you, want to spend time with you, and respect you.

·Personal Confidence: Projecting confidence in your language and behavior. This sounds obvious, but it's the greatest key to seduction. Projecting confidence is essential in any aspect or situation of your daily life.

·Adaptability: Being flexible and adaptable to different situations. Like a chameleon that survives by adapting in the hostile environment of the wild, as a seducer, it works the same. You'll need to adapt to comfortable situations as well as uncomfortable ones, always bringing out your best version and deriving the greatest benefit from each situation.

Practical Example: In your daily life, you decide to approach situations with a positive attitude. This not only improves your interactions with colleagues and friends but also makes you more attractive in different contexts.

Exercise: For a week, focus on addressing everyday situations with a positive attitude. Observe how it influences your interactions and how others perceive you.

Goal: Enhance your daily environment with an optimistic perspective.

The point of this chapter has been to make you see that seduction is not only useful for seducing women but also for any aspect of life, as explained in each previous point. Knowing this, I hope you understand that seduction is an art that you must practice day by day, in any aspect of your daily life. By doing this, you will build better relationships, be perceived as a high-value person, and gain respect. Applying seduction in your daily life will also help you make the most of your daily interactions, achieving personal goals, whether it's making sales or getting more favors from the people around you.

BE AWARE OF THE SEDUCTION TRAP

CHAPTER XXI

You've read it right, dear reader, seduction can and often is very addictive, which is something to be careful about. Once you start to have success in the field of seduction and see that you're starting to be successful with the female gender, you'll want more and it will become increasingly difficult to satisfy yourself.

What I mean by this is that you'll dedicate a lot of time and energy to it, which can be dangerous because you'll stop doing important things to go out and seduce. I'm telling you this from experience. So you have to be very careful with this, or at least be aware of where all this can lead you. Because it's certain that there's nothing wrong with dedicating time to seduction, but when your life revolves around it, that's when it becomes dangerous and addictive. I tell you this as advice and a warning.

However, if you're just starting out, it's advisable to dedicate a lot of time to it, because otherwise you'll never be able to hone your social skills and seductive abilities. Because at the beginning, the more time you dedicate to it, the better, as with any art, this one also requires learning.

So dear master of seduction, don't forget to put everything you've learned in this book into practice, because otherwise, what you've learned will be useless. It's okay to study seduction to have clear ideas and principles, but unfortunately seduction is more practical than theoretical.

Therefore... Go out, enjoy, seduce, and keep learning!

And don't forget that this can be addictive, but I'm sure the pleasure you'll get from becoming a seducer will be indescribable. Here I say goodbye, I hope I've helped you and it's been a pleasure to share my knowledge with you.

Can You Do Me A Favor?

As an independent writer, I need to ask you a small favor, which for you may be just 3 seconds of your time, but for me, it means a lot as it will help me reach more readers and also improve the positioning of my book.

I only ask you to do me this favor if you genuinely feel that the book has truly helped you, that you have gained new knowledge you didn't have before, and that it has motivated you to become the seducer you've always wanted to be.

If you feel all of the above, it would mean a lot to me if you could leave an honest and sincere review. I prefer it to be a five-star review, but the most important thing is that it's honest.

So, if I have helped you with this reading, the only favor I ask of you is to help me with a review so that I can reach more readers.

Thank you very much, and I wish you much success in this wonderful world of seduction and social relationships!

Do You Require Further Personalized Assistance?

If you feel like you've gained enough from reading this book and you're ready to take action, I'm glad and I hope you can put what you've learned into practice.

However, if you feel like you need more personalized help to overcome your fears, blocks, and insecurities, you might be interested to know that I offer one-on-one mentoring sessions via video call. My goal is to unlock your mind, overcome your barriers, and help you become a seducer.

If you're interested, don't hesitate to contact me. I'll do my best to share my knowledge with you in the most effective way possible. I'd be happy to help you, and together we'll help you achieve your goals in the world of seduction.

For more information, send me an email at contacto@mentalidadseductora.com, where I can provide you with more detailed information about the mentoring program. And if you have any quick questions, feel free to ask. We're in touch. I'll be waiting to hear from you.

BOOKS BY THIS AUTHOR

Seductive Mindset: How To Flirt With Women

The Arte Of Loving For Men: Love, Relationships And Women.